FDA LD$_{50}$ Mandai
Cures From Ever

To Kill

A Rat

An Antiquated Approach for Finding a Cure

All the Best
J C Spencer
Proverbs 16:3

J C Spencer

When rats stop dying to get drugs approved, it will SAVE **US**
$Trillions and usher in an ERA of Life-Saving Medical RESULTS

In Memory of
Patricia Champion
1945 - 2016

The Trillion Dollar answer to our healthcare and economic problems is to have more people healthy. A healthy person, company, and nation will be more productive and save untold dollars in medical costs.

To Kill A Rat applies to what CAN BE in the new era of medicine and healthcare.

About the Author

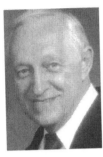

JC Spencer is the author of the Glycoscience Whitepaper and has written several Glycoscience books. He has studied the works of more than 700 M.D.s, PhDs, Scientists, Researchers, and Educators in the field of Glycoscience and brain function and collaborated with schools, universities, and research labs in thirteen countries. He has enjoyed international adventures and speaking engagements in many countries. Since the 1990s, he has worked closely with several specialists, doctors, and healthcare professionals in Glycoscience which resulted in the publishing of peer-reviewed papers evidencing improved brain function in Alzheimer's patients, and pilot surveys for various neurodegenerative challenges including Alzheimer's, Parkinson's, Huntington's, ALS, Lyme, Autism, and ADHD. He passionately envisions the field of QUANTUM GLYCOSCIENCE as the proven bull's eye, the Rosetta Stone, the Holy Grail, of medicine and of all healthcare.

JC Spencer is Founder and CEO of the TEXAS ENDOWMENT FOR MEDICAL RESEARCH, Inc, a 501(c)(3) faith-based medical research and education organization and think tank based in Houston, Texas. In collaboration with various organizations, he has conducted surveys on specific biological sugars throughout the United States, Canada, and some foreign countries. He has written extensively about Glycoscience and is also founder and CEO of the GLYCOSCIENCE INSTITUTE.

Mr Spencer and his wife, Karen, have four children, ten grandchildren and five great-grandchildren. They live in Houston, Texas.

Inquires for lecture bookings at universities, fund-raising, and other events, he may be reached at jcs@endowmentmed.org

During the last century, the focus has been
on problems instead of solutions. The medical
industry is focusing on treating the urgent
rather than addressing the important early on.

Drug companies know that the more critical the
problem, the greater the opportunity for profit.
The focus remains on sickness instead of wellness.

This is why we no longer need

The U.S. Department of Agriculture (USDA) compiles annual statistics on the number of animals including dogs, cats, primates, rabbits, hamsters and guinea pigs used in research in the United States. The Humane Society of the United States estimates that more than twenty-five million (25,000,000) vertebrate animals are used annually in research, testing, and education in the United States. This practice has continued for nearly a century. This book is not a campaign to save animals nor an effort to justify killing animals in the name of science; rather, it is a testament for how unnecessary is the FDA's LD_{50} mandate **To Kill A Rat**.

Credits

I am so very grateful for the many people who have contributed toward making possible **To Kill A Rat**. The work of over 700 MDs, PhDs, scientists, researchers, professors, and health professionals has contributed greatly to my understanding of Glycoscience. A special thanks to my mentors including H Reg McDaniel, MD, Bill McAnalley, PhD, Robert K Murray, MD, PhD, past faculties of doctors and professors, and a host of Glycoscience pioneers and Glycoscience enthusiast including Dr Ben Carson.

Charles Eschweiler, our director of research, has uncovered hidden knowledge by deep mining scientific literature and connecting the dots hidden from others.

Several friends assisted in proofing, editing, and making comments that made for significant improvement on my work and especially **To Kill A Rat**. Let me count the ways that Debra Hughes, MSN, RN helped make the book better. After it was "ready" to print she found 169 ways to make it better. Thank you Debra.

John Robert, worked along side me for nearly thirty years and our intellectual dialog grounded and encouraged me in ways that he never knew.

Thanks to our staff and past coworkers, those who have been in the background, friends, and family. These committed individuals have tolerated my obsession of living and breathing Glycoscience for all these years.

Karen Spencer, a leader of women and one husband - A big *"Thank You"* goes to my wife who has encouraged, corrected and edited much of my writings during the last twenty years. She too understands Glycoscience except the quantum part and has tolerated me for which I am grateful.

Jim Wing, loyal committed team leader, has served as our webmaster and assistant in so many ways including correcting my many articles and lessons over the years. Thanks Jim, for helping me so much with your tweaking of our publications, some of which have become a part of **To Kill A Rat**.

HL Champion, changer of lives, with family (Pat and Matthew). Thanks for being my confidante since 1980. Thanks for being co-founder and for serving as Vice President of the GLYCOSCIENCE INSTITUTE and the TEXAS ENDOWMENT FOR MEDICAL RESEARCH. Thanks partner. We dedicate this book to Patricia Champion (1945 - 2016) who served in the medical field for many years. Patricia was HL Champion's married partner for fifty years and assisted us in the founding of the GLYCOSCIENCE INSTITUTE. She was amazed and impressed with the outstanding health benefits the participants received in our Pilot Studies. It was an exciting journey for Pat to be with us for thirteen more years than the medical experts ever dreamed.

Nathan Gatch and team - Graphic Artist Cover Design. Thanks Nathan for your friendship over the years and for allowing me to help teach you photography forty some years ago. You and your wife, Lidia, have helped more than you know to further our work in Glycoscience.

Eddie Smith, more than a book publisher, consultant, mentor, coach, and friend for more than forty years.

Sources and References are listed at the end of sections or chapters.

Content

Chapter One

Chapter Two

Chapter Three

Chapter Four

Chapter Five

Chapter Six

Chapter Seven

Chapter Eight

Chapter Nine

Chapter Ten

Chapter Eleven

"Where there is no vision, the people perish..."
Proverbs 29:18a KJV

Foreword

"Reading this book will stimulate your neurons!" Those are the words of Robert K Murray, M.D., PhD in the Foreword of the Glycoscience textbook, Expand Your Mind - Improve Your Brain by JC Spencer.

The book you hold in your hand is designed to stimulate your neurons. To Kill A Rat applies to what CAN BE in the medical and healthcare field of America and the world. When your neurons are stimulated to do what they are designed to do, the lame walk, the deaf hear, and the blind see... no medical claim made or intended.

For more than twenty years I have has gained an understanding of what can be achieved through Glycoscience and faith and what will be achieved through this New Frontier of Medicine. I have participated with many M.D.s, PhDs, researchers and educators in several countries. I have also written reports on thousands of laboratory, anecdotal, and clinical results.

After founding The Endowment for Medical Research in Houston, Texas, we sponsored Glycoscience Medical Conferences. The major aims of these very successful and well attended Conferences was to educate healthcare workers and others of the new scientific area of Glycoscience and its possible application to helping individuals who suffer from chronic neurodegenerative conditions.

Robert K Murray said, *"JC Spencer is a man with tremendous energy, enthusiasm and commitment to the objective potential he sees in the field of Glycoscience. The readers of this book will find these and other qualities shine through as they peruse this significant work"*.

It is my desire for the reader to gain a better understanding and attain a deep caring spirit for the suffering of the millions with chronic neurodegenerative conditions.

Post Traumatic Stress ~~Disorder~~ (PTS~~D~~), Alzheimer's, dementia, Parkinson's, fetal alcohol syndrome and every other neurological challenge is caused by or accentuated by a misfolding of the proteins on the surface of human cells. We have learned through Glycoscience how to better fold the proteins. When improper folding occurs in the brain, it results in a lack of cognitive malfunction.

Knowledge of the nutritional damage that sugars and sweeteners on the human body has blinded many scientists and researchers from seeing the beneficial sugars the body requires. The study of these various sugars is Glycoscience and the author coined the expression, "Smart Sugars."

My studies and experiences covering more than two decades have uncovered a myriad of fascinating research concerning neurons. I understands that our medical systems and all healthcare will benefit greatly when we better understand neurons and neurotransmitters. My studies include optimal nutrition for the brain and a host of relevant matters on basic psychology, savants, mental exercises and recovery from brain damage.

With my fellow pioneers in Glycoscience, we have learned the benefits of a variety of collaborating disciplines that include pH, electrolytes, rogue electrons, mitochondria, and nutrition to name a few.

The TEXAS ENDOWMENT FOR MEDICAL RESEARCH in 2017 obtained a licensing agreement for intellectual properties and technologies of earlier works from my earlier works that are consolidated with works from other organizations.

The Sugar Pill has no credibility and is called, "placebo". But... wait.

I grew up listening to Paul Harvey on the radio. He would refer to the United States by saying, "*US – that's us.*" So, in the book, I may refer to the United States in the enduring term, "US."

Introduction

The "Sugar Pill"

The "Sugar Pill" used as a placebo indicates just how worthless is regular sugar. However, there is a beneficial category of biological sugars known as "Smart Sugars" found in nature to save and extend your life. Who would have thought that the sugar has the potential to solve some of our greatest health problems?

Smart Sugars are destined to take US to a better future. These sugars can provide healthier children and stressless parents. Studies verify that these special sugars can support neurological function for those with PTSD, MS, ALS, Parkinson's, Alzheimer's, Huntington's, Stroke, and other nerve function.

The special sugars are the building blocks for glycoforms. Glycoforms are glycan and glycoprotein signal receptor sites on the surface of your cells. Glycolipids operate inside your cells.

What Are Smart Sugars?

These Smart Sugars are operating this moment in your body as your cellular Operating System (OS). Their responsibility is to process all DNA data communication to function, maintain, repair, and replicate. These sugars actually give LIFE to your blood.

Glycoscience (glyco is Greek for sugar) has been hidden in plain sight and is now revealed to radically change how we live. Glycoscience IS the New Frontier of Medicine. This emerging technology will make a major difference in human health. It will do so because the sugars instigate an aggressive attack on viral infections and resistant bacteria.

Big Pharma and our government have already invested billions of dollars in Glycoscience and the general public is still in the dark.

Knowledge of Glycoscience is young. The term "glycobiology" was coined at Oxford University in 1988.

Early in the 21st century, the science of sugars was reconsidered by the

National Academy of Sciences, the top scientific governmental body in Washington, DC. This prestigious group is made up of Nobel Prize winners and those nominated by Nobel Prize winners.

A distinguished panel of glycoscientists was commissioned for a collaborative effort to explore the future of Glycoscience. The National Research Council drew from the National Academies: the National Academy of Sciences, National Academy of Engineering, Institute of Medicine. The project was supported by National Institutes of Health, the National Science Foundation, U.S. Department of Energy, the Food and Drug Administration, and the Howard Hughes Medical Institute. Together, they were commissioned to develop the roadmap for the future of Glycoscience. By the close of 2012, the panel published its 200 page report *Transforming Glycoscience - A Road Map for the Future*. Here, they went on record, stating that:

> *"Glycans impact the structure/function of every living cell in humans, animals, and plants."*

The Academy expanded on the importance of the sugars, saying:

> *"Glycans play roles in almost every biological process and are involved in every major disease"*
> and
> *"Elimination of any single class of glycans from an organism results in death."*

Another indication of the importance of Glycoscience is found in the bowels of the National Library of Medicine where almost 700,000 references point to research already conducted on some of the most significant life changing biological sugars. The majority of these papers were published within the last few years.

Immunological Testing Instead of Toxicity Testing

Toxins damage the cellular Operating System (OS) and render it dysfunctional in its ability to properly process data. Toxins alter gene expression and corrupt the body's function to properly maintain, replicate, and repair cells, tissue, and vital organs.

Immunological testing instead of toxicity testing will safely and naturally cover the whole spectrum. Immunity is lowered by the very presence of toxins and renders unnecessary the need to test for toxins.

During the past two decades, I have worked with or studied the work of more than 700 MDs, PhDs, Scientists, Researchers and Educators in the field of GLYCOSCIENCE and Brain Function. During this period I have observed "impossible" ailments disappear that standard medical practices cannot address. These catastrophic ailments disappeared through immunology – the modulation of the human immune system. The modulation of the immune system was observed when "Smart Sugars" were supplemented into the human diet.

In this book, I present an outline of some of the health benefits we have discovered in collaborative efforts with universities in several countries. We have tested the safety and clinical efficacy of certain biological sugars and evidence for the last two decades. The results conclude that several trillions of dollars can be saved through application of Glycoscience.

For example, American veterans can lead the way by example for fewer dollars producing greater results. Using toxin free biological Smart Sugars can help relieve human suffering in thousands if not millions of PTSD suffers.

During the last century, the focus has been on problems instead of solutions. The medical complex is focused to resolve the urgent instead of addressing the important early on. Big Pharma knows that the more critical the problem, the greater the opportunity for profit. The focus remains on sickness instead of wellness.

The Truths in this book are self-evident!

Doctors were once held to high esteem.
Doctors can again be held to High Esteem.

The information you hold in your hand will SAVE HUMAN LIVES, can SAVE US Trillions of dollars, and millions of rats.

Chapter One

"Do No Harm"
Can Again Be The Rule

The Food and Drug Administration 's LD_{50} Rule

"Do no harm!" was the medical battle cry that was lost to toxic drugs. The FDA has a procedure that blocks any safe toxin free cure from approval to reach the market. The FDA will not even allow water to have a medical claim that it treats dehydration. The antiquated FDA procedure is called LD_{50}. The lethal dose standard was established to verify how toxic a medicine is by determining how much it takes to kill fifty percent (50%) of the animals in a study. Any medicine that kills less than 50% is not eligible for FDA approval.

When non-toxic is a toxin

The entanglement of what is and what is not is often so confusing that the public believes the opposite of what is or what is not. A Deception is the twin brother of A Lie.

For years, I thought if something was labeled non-toxic that it was toxin free. When I was told that was not the case, I could not believe it. The definition of "toxic" is a substance that can produce personal injury or illness to humans when inhaled, swallowed, or absorbed through the skin. There are highly toxic, less toxic, and non-toxic. But, if you have a bunch of healthy rats and only 49% are killed by a product — that product can be labeled non-toxic and the company would not be in violation of the law. According to the federal regulatory definition, non-toxic doesn't necessarily mean "no toxins at all" or "absolutely safe". Start looking for the label "Toxin free" which is a term reserved for products that are proven to contain no toxins. But, I digress.

The LD_{50} test was adopted in 1927 and has ever since continued to be tested on animals, usually laboratory mice. Animal testing is illegal in much of the world and resistance is growing against the unreliable archaic LD_{50}

requirement. In 2011, the FDA began to inch away from the mandatory LD_{50} method. The first drug to bypass animal testing consisted of botulinum neurotoxins found in the cosmetic drug Botox.

Origin of the FDA

The Federal Food and Drugs Act was passed into law in 1906. The origins of the FDA, according to their website is traced back to 1862 when President Lincoln appointed chemist Charles M. Wetherill to head the Chemical Division in the new U. S. Department of Agriculture.

A brief history continues, *"In the following decade Wetherill's successor as chief chemist of the USDA, Peter Collier, began working on the ubiquitous problem of food adulteration. Harvey W. Wiley replaced Collier in 1883, leading the division as it grew into the Bureau of Chemistry in 1901. The bureau was charged to enforce the first comprehensive federal statute of its kind, the Federal Food and Drugs Act, when that law was passed in 1906.*

"In 1927 Congress authorized the formation of the Food, Drug, and Insecticide Administration from the regulatory wing of the Bureau of Chemistry; the name of the agency was shortened to the Food and Drug Administration in 1930. [The] FDA left the Department of Agriculture in 1940 for the Federal Security Agency [FSA], which was created a year earlier. In 1953 [the] FDA joined the Department of Health, Education, and Welfare [HEW] after Congress established that department to assume certain functions of FSA. In 1968 the agency became part of the Public Health Service within HEW. "When the education function was removed from HEW to create a separate department, HEW became the Department of Health and Human Services in 1980.

"[The] FDA's responsibilities derive from statutes that date back to the early twentieth century. Harvey Wiley fought long and hard to unify disparate interest groups behind a federal law to deal with serious problems in the food and drug supply. Through Wiley's crusading, the support of the General Federation of Women's Clubs, the work of muckraking journalists, the efforts of state and local food and drug officials, cooperation from the American Medical Association (AMA) and

the American Pharmaceutical Association (APA), *the impact of Upton Sinclair's The Jungle, [a novel depicting the filth of the meat packing industry]. Congress approved one of the landmarks of Progressive era legislation in 1906, the Food and Drugs Act. Among other provisions, this law charged the Bureau of Chemistry to control--albeit to a lesser extent than Wiley and others had hoped--adulterated and misbranded drugs and food in interstate commerce.*

"[The] FDA initiated a movement to replace the problematical aspects of the 1906 act during the nascent New Deal. Again, the support of women's groups, journalists, and others was important to the final passage of a bill, as was the repercussion from a toxic preparation of the wonder drug, sulfanilamide. So-called Elixir Sulfanilamide employed an untested solvent for the drug, diethylene glycol, and eventually it killed over a hundred people, most of whom were children. The 1938 Food, Drug, and Cosmetic Act, which remains the basic law we have today, featured many provisions lacking in the 1906 Act. For example, it mandated that all new drugs be proved safe before marketing, therapeutic devices and cosmetics become subject to regulation, and standards of identity and quality be instituted for foods. The law also formalized [The] FDA's ability to conduct factory inspections.

"Over the following decades numerous amendments and other acts broadened [the] FDA's responsibilities considerably. These include a mandate for agency testing of insulin and antibiotics; regulation of chemical pesticides and food and color additives; distinction between prescription and nonprescription medications; regulation of drug efficacy; ensuring of good manufacturing practices; control of prescription drug advertising; regulation of therapeutic agents of biological origin; and oversight of nutrition labeling. The realities of enforcing such broad statutes requires [the]FDA's interaction with a variety of political, economic, and social interests. Today, as in the past, [the] FDA strives above all else to safeguard the health and well being of the American people."

FDA Whistleblowers on Corruptions and Fraud

Whistleblowers and investigators within and without the FDA have made strong accusations about wrong doings over the years. These accusations have ranged in serious coverups of the harm certain drugs have to agents ownership of stock on drugs companies for which they were authorized to approve drugs. To follow the money reveals these serious accusations.

Fraud has been known to abound both ways. Fraud lawsuits often involve drug companies that promote or encourage doctors to prescribe drugs for off-label uses, give doctors kickbacks to prescribe certain medications, or fail to comply with the FDA's manufacturing and safety regulations.

The system is far from perfect. It is easy to violate the Health Insurance Portability and Accountability Act (HIPAA)'s Privacy Rules. With advanced storage of data, perhaps nothing is safely stored. Whistleblowers and attorneys have exemption from HIPAA's Privacy Rules. Data and activities may be shared with an attorney, health oversight agency or public health authority. This type of information can demonstrate intent to commit fraud or actual instances of fraud.

Federal law prohibits drug companies from offering doctors any form of compensation in exchange for prescribing their drugs. It is reported to be commonplace for pharmaceutical companies to provide doctors with free golf outings, tickets to wine-tasting events, and paid speaking arrangements in exchange for prescribing certain drugs.

Adulteration fraud is the altering of a drug outside the rules of current Good Manufacturing Practice (GMP) regulations. GMP regulations are to assure that a drug is safe for use and has the quality and purity characteristics that the drug is represented to contain.

Clinical trial fraud is when a pharmaceutical company submits false data to the FDA to receive approval of a new drug. The drug company can be liable for fraud if it fails to include clinical trial data regarding the negative side effects of a new drug or minimizes the severity or frequency of these side effects.

In 2012, the Government Accountability Project publicly denounced the FDA's implementation of a surveillance system against employees trying to blow the whistle on critical safety issues.

Acting Commissioner of the FDA, Stephen Ostroff, M.D, issued a whistleblower protection memo to all FDA employees on January 4, 2016.

DEPARTMENT OF HEALTH & HUMAN SERVICES
Public Health Service
Food and Drug Administration

Memorandum   Date: January 4, 2016
From: Acting Commissioner of Food and Drugs
Subject: Whistleblower Protection and NO FEAR Act Policy Statement

To: All FDA Employees

The Food and Drug Administration (FDA) has established itself as an agency that upholds its strict code of conduct with exacting standards. For this reason, I strongly support the Whistleblower Protection Act (WPA) of 1989 and the Whistleblower Protection Enhancement Act (WPEA) of 2012, which affords employees the legal protection to report allegations of official wrongdoing without fear of reprisal. Under the WPA and WPEA, employees and applicants are entitled to all the protection which prohibits retaliation for reporting waste, fraud, and abuse. This law preserves the integrity and high standards of the scientific processes that guide our agency. The FDA further supports the rights of all employees to engage in protected activity under current civil rights statutes and Executive Orders.

The U.S. Office of Special Counsel is empowered to administer an impartial and effective complaint management process to address complaints of whistleblower retaliation for most of the Executive Branch, including the FDA. Reprisal against individuals will not be tolerated for disclosure of information in which the employee believes there is reasonable belief of violation of any law, rule or regulation; gross mismanagement; gross waste of funds; abuse of authority; or a substantial and specific danger to public health or safety. Reprisal for whistleblowing includes taking or failing to take, or threatening to take a personal action with respect to any employee because of a protected disclosure of information.

Employees may report allegations of reprisal for whistleblowing to the Office of the Special Counsel at https://osc.gov/ or contact them on 1-800-

872-9855. Employees may also raise such allegations to the Health and Human Services' Office of the Inspector General at www.oig.hhs.gov or contact them at 1 -800- 447-8477.

The Notification and Federal Employee Antidiscrimination and Retaliation (NO FEAR) Act of 2002 mandates that all Federal employees must be trained concerning their rights and protections under the antidiscrimination and whistleblower laws within ninety (90) days of their entrance into the Federal government and every two years thereafter. The FDA offers an on-line training course for new hires and current employees. Please take the time to learn more about your rights and responsibilities under these important laws.

This memorandum supersedes the memorandum from the Commissioner of Food and Drugs dated May 5, 2014 to all FDA employees.

Stephen Ostroff, M.D

Reports of Times When Doctors Strike

It is a disputed report that during a one-month strike by physicians in 1976 in Los Angeles County the death rate dropped by 18 percent. This may have been due because many elective surgeries were postponed.

Following a 1983 four-month Israeli doctor's strike, a study of public perception showed 25% of the people surveyed believed the strike had resulted in major health problems. However, there was a reported connection between the doctors' strike and fewer deaths.

In 1984, a doctor's strike in Varkaus, Finland, simply resulted in fewer visits for minor ailments. The public apparently had no significant harmful effects and were glad when the doctors returned to work.

Again, in Israel in 2000, the death rate dropped considerably when physicians in public hospitals implemented the strike. The connection of fewer deaths during the withdrawal of medical services was substantiated by a survey of burial societies. The Jerusalem Post survey showed that the number of funerals dropped drastically during that time period. The month of May one area recorded 93 funerals compared to 153 in May 1999. Other areas were close to this decline in deaths.

It is my opinion that the main cause for the decline in deaths is the decline in drug use. However, Avi Yisraeli, director general of the Hadassah Medical Organization, offered his explanation. *"Mortality is not the only measure of harm to health. Lack of medical intervention can lead to disability, pain, and reduced functioning. Elective surgery can bring about a great improvement in a patient's condition, but it can also mean disability and death in the weakest patients. And patients who do not undergo diagnosis or surgery now could decline or die in a few months due to the postponement."*

Research Scientists are in Panic

Research scientists are in panic over possible lack of funding. And yet, we are entering a new era of medical science breakthroughs.

After the UK and US voting results, scientists are fearful of losing research funding. Most funding in the UK comes through the EU. British researchers were soon removed from research grant application list because of Brexit.

In the last hours of 2016, Scientific American's Dana Hunter, showing disdain toward President Trump, blogged, *"Our scientific endeavors are under severe threat... Science is going to need our help to survive this regime. We used to be the scientific leaders of the world. If we want to stay in the forefront of scientific advances, we will need to resist Trump and his merry band of anti-science lackeys at every turn."*

The new US administration's positions on science may restore fiscal sanity in Washington by focusing on self-evident results instead of simply hurling more money at bad science. The public is tired of hearing the same battle cry made by President Richard Nixon, *"We'll find a cure in ten years."*

Instead of just caring for people with debilitating diseases, we cure people through a toxin free approach that demands the FDA take the handcuffs off scientists and remove the deadly bureaucracy that costs trillions of dollars.

Our Texas Senator, Ted Cruz is quoted as saying, *"We need to tear down the barriers blocking a new era of medical innovation, and the primary inhibitor is the government itself. Its past time to unleash a supply-side medical revolution, so that instead of simply caring for people with debilitating diseases, we cure them. ... we need to modernize the FDA's approach, expand the Accelerating Medicines Partnership, and embrace a culture of innovation."*

New knowledge replaces old theories. New technologies enable us to discover, verify, and integrate Glycoscience findings which open doors to tomorrow's toxin free functional medicine/foods.

Private Research Platform

Private research and development will streamline science projects and eliminate much of the red tape bureaucracy. Glycoscience is, without question, the future of medicine and healthcare and will usher in an era of Life Saving Medical RESULTS,

Source and References:

https://www.ncbi.nlm.nih.gov/pmc/articles/PMC1127364/

https://blogs.scientificamerican.com/rosetta-stones/troubling-signs-for-science-under-trump/?WT.mc_id=SA_DD_20161227

https://royalsociety.org/science-events-and-lectures/2016/11/evolutionary-biology/

http://Glycosciencewhitepaper.com

Expand Your Mind - Improve Your Brain
http://endowmentmed.org/content/view/826/106/

Change Your Sugar, Change Your Life
http://DiabeticHope.com

Glycoscience Lesson #49   http://GlycoscienceNEWS.com/pdf/Lesson49.pdf

http://EzineArticles.com/?expert=JC_Spencer

© The Endowment for Medical Research

http://endowmentmed.org

There are government costs and family costs.
In the end, all the costs come from the family.

Treating PTSÐ costs the VA 5 time more
than those without PTSÐ.

$100 Billion here
and $100 Billion there
soon adds up!

Chapter Two

Trillion Dollar
Savings Examples

One example for saving US a Trillion Dollars per year.

"Delaying the onset of Alzheimer's for 15 million patients just one year could result in a national savings of $1.125 trillion minus normal living costs, still leaving a savings of approximately $1 trillion."

Research show that the same basic procedure also delays the onset of ALS (amyotrophic laterals sclerosis aka Lou Gehrig's)

One Smart Sugar Trehalose

Link to the Alzheimer's Mystery
New Research Confirms How
This Method Delays Alzheimer's

A research team at the University of Bonn, Germany has discovered that the sugar Trehalose goes beyond just reducing the secretion of the neurotoxic amyloid β-peptide within the brain. Previous research indicates that amyloid β peptide is the crucial step in the development of Alzheimer's.

The University of Bonn research paper published March 8, 2016 explains how Alzheimer's progression is slowed. Trehalose is found to alter the metabolism of the Alzheimer related amyloid precursor protein. Cell treatment with Trehalose decreased the degradation of full-length amyloid precursor protein and its cell terminal fragments. Biochemical and cell biological experiments revealed that Trehalose also alters the subcellular distribution.

The Journal of Alzheimer's Disease in early 2013 published a paper of the research performed by the Miami Miller School of Medicine and presented through the University of Miami. The university study was inspired by two very encouraging Alzheimer's Pilot Surveys conducted by The Endowment for Medical Research in Houston and published in <u>Proceedings</u> of the Fisher Institute for Medical Research in March 2006 and March 2007.

In 2008, I wrote these words in the textbook on Glycoscience and brain function, Expand Your Mind - Improve Your Brain, *"The economical impact this discovery can have on the nation is astounding. There are currently some six million Alzheimer's patients in the United States with an expected fifteen million within the next few years. The current cost of caring for these victims is estimated at $75,000 per person year per year. That is an annual economic burden of four hundred and fifty billion dollars.*

"Delaying the onset of Alzheimer's for 15 million patients just one year could result in a national savings of $1.125 trillion minus normal living costs, still leaving a savings of approximately $1 trillion."

Abstract from University of Bonn:

Trehalose alters subcellular trafficking and the metabolism of the Alzheimer-associated amyloid precursor protein.

J Biol Chem 2016 Mar 8. Epub 2016 Mar 8.
Nguyen T Tien, Ilker Karaca, Irfan Y Tamboli, Jochen Walter

The disaccharide trehalose is commonly considered to stimulate autophagy. Cell treatment with trehalose could decrease cytosolic aggregates of potentially pathogenic proteins, including mutant huntingtin, alpha-synuclein and phosphorylated tau that are associated with neurodegenerative diseases. Here, we demonstrate that trehalose also alters the metabolism of the Alzheimer related amyloid precursor protein (APP).

Cell treatment with trehalose decreased the degradation of full-length APP and its C-terminal fragments (CTFs). Trehalose also reduced the secretion of the amyloid β-peptide. Biochemical and cell biological experiments revealed that trehalose alters the subcellular distribution and decreases the degradation of APP-CTFs in endolysosomal compartments. Trehalose also led to strong accumulation of the autophagic marker proteins LC3-II and p62, and decreased the proteolytic activation of the lysosomal hydrolase cathepsin D. The combined data indicate that trehalose decreases the lysosomal metabolism of APP by alterating its endocytic vesicular transport.

Affiliation: University of Bonn, Germany jochen.walter@ukb.uni-bonn.de.
(End of Abstract)

Source and References:

University of Bonn   http://ncbi.nlm.nih.gov/pubmed/22976077

University of Miami   http://endowmentmed.org/pdf/SmartLesson89.pdf

Expand Your Mind - Improve Your Brain   http://endowmentmed.org/content/view/826/106/

Change Your Sugar, Change Your Life   http://DiabeticHope.com

Glycoscience Lesson #41   http://GlycoscienceNEWS.com/pdf/Lesson41.pdf

http://EzineArticles.com/?expert=JC_Spencer

© **The Endowment for Medical Research**   http://endowmentmed.org

Chapter Three and Four is an Overview of the LIFE Giving Aspects of Glycoscience

Excerpts are from the Glycoscience Whitepaper and the Glycoscience Workbook from the GLYCOSCIENCE INSTITUTE

Chapter Three

LIFE Giving Glycoscience
The Past & Present
of Medicine and Healthcare

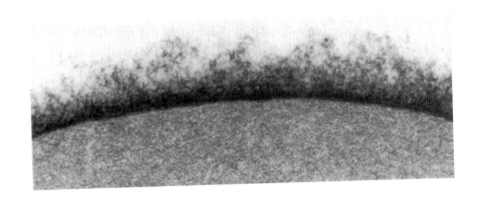

Glycan / Glycoproteins on the surface of a red blood cell. These Glycoforms transmit and receive all cellular signals for the human body.

"Why have you not heard about this before?"

Glycoscience will soon be taught in all
university and high school science classes.
And, will be integrated into mainstream medicine.

Glycobiology

The term "glycobiology" was coined in 1988 at Oxford University.

Glycobiology is the foundational branch of Glycoscience that studies the essential sugars that are the building blocks of glycoforms.

Glycobiology explains that Cellular Communication is the key to all life.

Sugars are carbohydrates. Many carbohydrates are not good for your health. But, several specific sugars are so beneficial that they are essential to LIFE. They are at work in your body every moment. I call them Smart Sugars.

Glycans are links of specific sugar molecules.

DNA and proteins are formed by templates, while glycans are formed more from environmental influences. The cell's environmental factors contribute to each unique glycan design, as varied as fingerprints. These known and unknown factors provide each glycan with properties that are more complex and difficult to study and duplicate than genes.

Glycoproteins are links of specific protein with sugar molecules.

Specific glycans are attached to specific proteins. Structure and function are influenced by the DNA and cell environmental needs. Alignment of the glycans with the proteins determines cell function including blood type.

Glycolipids are links of specific sugar and lipid molecules:

Glycolipids provide cellular recognition and energy to help maintain membrane stability. This enables cells to attach to other cells to form tissue. Lipids contain hydrocarbons, the cellular building blocks for structure and function. Glycolipids are composed mostly of non-protein cell membrane.

Glycans are the key to processing all communication and we are hardwired for...truth and perfection. Our cells are ever attempting to achieve purity by continuing to dump toxins out of the body.

Communication makes everything happen.

Cell Communication
Your LIFE started by communication even before you were conceived

In the beginning, you were a cell; yes, you were two cells. The sperm from the father and egg from the mother were coated with a sophisticated communication system. They came into agreement when the sperm impregnated the egg. The two cells became one. Signals from the egg were immediately switched to a new message proclaiming to other sperm, *"Leave me alone. It's too late - I'm taken."* The two cells became one... a stem cell. Your life began.

Your original stem cell began to divide and manufacture more stem cells and produce differential cells to create every organ and designated part of your body.

Tens of Millions of Dollars are Invested into Learning How Cells Communicate

Here is but one example:

Announcement was made October 6, 2011 that researchers hope to learn how cells communicate. Using this information, researchers hope that cells that cause human neurological and other diseases can be manipulated.

New discoveries in glycomics build upon all that we already know. Knowing what to do with this data is the key. We do not need new drugs to manipulate cells. We need Smart Sugars to LET the cells communicate like they were designed. This is accomplished by the glycoprotein receptor sites which are made from these sugars. The glycoprotein coating of cells somewhat like fuzz on a peach or trees on the earth make up the Operating System (OS), the communication system of the body. This is how the DNA codes are read and processed.

The $10 million grant by the National Institutes of Health (NIH) is awarded to the University of Nevada, Reno and the University of Nevada School of Medicine for research into how cells communicate.

Personal follow-up from this $10 million NIH investment is inconclusive; however, in 2016 the University of Nevada School of Medicine's Department of Psychiatry were scheduling research with schizophrenia individuals and stem cells.

We have documented proliferation of an individual's own stem cells is achieved then certain specific Smart Sugars are used to glycosylate the cells. Proliferation of stem cells in an individual's body is paramount to improved health and glycosylation and improved cell signals is the pathway to make that happen.

Much of my writings and classes explore various aspects of Glycoscience and how cells communicate.

New Scientist, 10/02 reported, "'*This is going to be the future,*' declares biochemist Gerald Hart of Johns Hopkins University in Baltimore. '*We won't understand immunology, neurology, developmental biology or disease until we get a handle on glycobiology.*' ... '*If you ask, what is the glycome for a single cell type, it's probably many thousands of times more complex than the genome,*' says Ajit Varki, Director of the Glycobiology Research and Training Center at the University of California in San Diego ... Raymond Dwek, Head of the University of Oxford's Glycobiology Institute, who coined the term "*glycobiology*" in 1988, says that sugars were often dismissed as unimportant, '*as just decorations on proteins - people didn't know how to deal with them.*" They could not have been more wrong.

As recent advances in genetics have unfolded, the importance of sugars has become ever more apparent ... Varki sees it as a journey of exploration. '*It's like we've just discovered the continent of North America. Now we have to send out scouting parties to find out how big it is ...*'

Many participants eating phytosugars (plant sugars), in our nutritional pilot surveys, not only experienced improved cognitive abilities, but also experienced overall general health and well being. If you are starting to replace your regular table sugar, we would appreciate your completing a general health evaluation form which you can request or download from our website at http://endowmentmed.org

While the science of glycobiology is relatively new it was not called as such until 1988. Some research in the US on glycoproteins and other sugar-containing molecules was conducted prior to 1980. In 1985 a research group at Oxford published a paper in *Nature* about glycosylation. Oxford University Press in 1988 started the journal *Glycobiology*. It was Raymond Dwek, Head of the University of Oxford's Glycobiology Institute, who actually coined the term *"glycobiology"* in 1988, and it was soon used in science around the world.

The following is a quote from the Institute for Glycomics at Griffith University: *"Glycomics is the study of applied biology and chemistry that deals with the structure and function of carbohydrates (sugars). The term glycomics is derived from the chemical prefix for sweetness or a sugar, 'glyco', and was formed to follow the naming convention established by genomics (which deals with genes) and proteomics (which deals with proteins)."*

Generating the Electricity to Power the Signals

Electrolytes play a major role in neuron conductivity. Your body contains a very sophisticated battery to power all of its functions including thought. When you feel "run down," that is exactly what has happened. Your battery is low. Without electrolytes, you could not move, think, or live.

Electrolytes are in a gel or liquid of salts that conduct electricity. These salts are made up of certain minerals including calcium, chloride, magnesium, potassium, and sodium ions, which are essential for the flow of electrons and, of course, good human health. Because electrolytes are essential minerals, they cannot be substituted in the diet with anything less. These minerals are absolutely vital. The absence of these minerals results in poor communication and a flawed immune system.

The Smart Sugars control switches more sophisticated than just off and on switches – some are dimmer switches that fade in and out to regulate the current and signal flow. These dimmer switches are responsible for dividing cells.

Research shows the sugar O-Linked β-*N*-acetylglucosamine (O-GlcNAc) plays a role in cell division. N-Acetylglucosamine (N-acetyl-D-glucosamine, or GlcNAc) is a monosaccharide derivative of glucose and one of the building blocks for glycoproteins. It is an amide between glucosamine and acetic acid. Understanding these newly discovered sugar switches reveals that the cellular circuitry is much more complex than previously thought. GlcNAc is generally not elongated or modified to form the more complex sugar structures. O-GlcNAc is attached and removed multiple times in the life of a polypeptide, often cycling rapidly and at different rates at different sites on a polypeptide.

The chemical changes act more like "dimmer" switches than simple on/off switches. The communication between O-GlcNAc and phosphorylation is a paradigm-shift in terms of signaling. So says Gerald Hart, PhD director of biological chemistry at Johns Hopkins School of Medicine. He added, *"I think of phosphorylation as a micro-switch that regulates the circuitry of cell division, and O-GlcNAcylation as the safety switch that regulates the microswitches."*

Authors of the paper:

Johns Hopkins authors on the paper are Zihao Wang, Chad Slawson, Kaoru Sakabe, Win D. Cheung and Gerald W. Hart. Other authors are Namrata D. Udeshi, Philip D. Compton, Jeffrey Shabanowitz and Donald F. Hunt, all of the University of Virginia.

Source and References:

http://www.sciencedaily.com/releases/2010/02/100205112105.htm

http://endowmentmed.org

Your Operating System

The wonders of your first stem cell contained your complete blueprint from all your ancestors back to the first couple. The RNA confirms that one woman was the mother of the human race. The operating systems of super computers cannot compare to the complexity of design of the operating system (OS) of your body.

Using your DNA as the blueprint, it is estimated that a few trillion new cells are manufactured in the body every day. When the OS of your computer becomes corrupted, your computer becomes dysfunctional. Likewise, when the OS of your body becomes faulty, your DNA processes errors that produce corrupted unhealthy cells.

Smart Sugars Help Transcribe Your DNA

New technology allows us to view damaged DNA closeup. Today, with powerful electron microscopes we can zoom into the human cell where we are learning disease causes. The scientific study of health vs. sickness has been viewed from afar for centuries. We are beginning to solve the mystery of the signals of inner and outer cellular communication. The glycolipids (inner cellular) and the Glycoproteins (outer cellular) ARE the OS for the human body. We are learning that when we improve the OS, we improve brain and body performance. This is the function of Smart Sugars.

Functional sugars have influenced the health of the human body all along (how the different sugars are used) but we did not understand glycosylation. Today, the positive functions of these sugars are becoming more self-evident, better documented, and certainly better understood. The ability to better study sick and healthy molecules and to look into the cell is enabling non-orthodocs and research scientists to see solutions outside mainstream drug use.

Nanoparticles, be they proper nutrients or deadly toxins, nudge and sometimes lunge us toward health or sickness. This new understanding of glycomics and toxins will forever alter the way we live. The improvements in healthcare may not happen through "push" or "force." It is the vacuum of need that is seeking out whatever works. Does anyone have a natural deficiency of drugs made from coal tar? But, everyone has a natural deficiency of nutrients and the one you need the most will perform the most benefit.

My father taught me to take care of the little things in life and the big things will take care of themselves. I never realized the true significance of that wisdom until I learned about the cell. But the cell is large in size compared to atoms, electrons, and ions. Position of everything affects function.

Chromosomes occupy exact positions within the cell. Scientists have discovered the location of genes within the nucleus of the cell and how these positions vary in relationship to the condition of the cell. When the genes move within the nucleus they profoundly influence the health of the cell.

The genome orchestrates the symphony of life from cell-to-cell. This orchestration influences cell division and the health of new cells. German cell scientist, Theodor Boveri, nearly twenty years ago, called the regions within the cells, "chromosome territories." But only recently have we been able to see them with new 3-D imaging technology and chromosome fluorescent markers viewed by microscopy.

The propensity for specific chromosomes to reside in a distinct region of the cell next to other specific chromosomes has profound health significance and influences a gene to turn off or on. This obviously affects the cell function and transcription of the DNA for cell division.

As human activity changes, so does the arrangement of the chromosomes. Vital food in the form of nano-nutrients, sugars, and specific trace minerals cause electrical and chemical reactions. The nutrients and toxins trigger the gene. But something else happens. Other related genes on nearby chromosomes respond in synchronized response like birds taking flight. This is somewhat like the synapses in the brain we have written about and now we see similar orchestrations of genes within the cell.

Glycomics and genomics are shining lights in the field of medical science.

These lights are a blinding force in the dark age of that region of medical science that limits itself to drug use and abuse. Royal Sugars are the ingredients for tomorrow's healthcare system. The number of physicians integrating sugars into their practices is growing because they are witnessing remarkable results almost regardless of what is wrong with their patients. Maybe treating the symptom has not been the solution. Understanding the cause and using an ounce of prevention is worth a pound of cure. Some doctors are saying that simply improving the OS is providing cures. More research is needed and universities around the world are looking into Smart Sugars even though that research is normally not funded by the drug cartels. The Massachusetts Institute of Technology (MIT) was right. Glycomics will [continue to] change the way we live. We have some exciting fresh out of the lab research to give you in future Smart Sugar lessons.

* Royal Sugars was the term used earlier. Today, we call them, "Smart Sugars."

Source and References:

http://www.endowmentmed.org/pdf/SmartLesson9.pdf

Even Your DNA Requires Sugar in its Construction

Supporting Neurodegenerative Repair with Smart Sugars

In the book, Expand Your Mind - Improve Your Brain, I discussed regeneration of tissue. In an article entitle, *Supporting Evidence Links Glycomics to Neurodegenerative Repair*. We covered a News Report out of Dublin, Ireland that supported our own findings about glycoscience and cell damage repair and neural degeneration and repair. The book "Neural Degeneration and Repair: Gene Expression Profiling, Proteomics and Systems Biology" was touted as the first book linking glycomics and nerve cell damage repair.. The book is selling for $113 EU which is about $175 US. Well, it is not quite the first book to link glycomics to neurodegenerative repair. In Expand Your Mind - Improve Your Brain, I cover an analysis of Nerve Cell Damage and Repair using Genomics, Transcriptomics, Proteomics, Glycomics and Systems Biology.

In 2009 we reported that the sugar Trehalose and an enzyme was used in spine repair. I quote myself, *"Neurological challenges of all kinds can be overcome IF the neutransmitters are connected or re-connected properly. Blocking of neurons can be protein plaque buildup. Nerve cells may not communicate because of protein buildup as scar tissue that inhibits nerve fiber regeneration. The ability to sprout new axons or nerve fibers can regain nerve function even in spinal cord injuries. Trehalose has been known to help control inflammation and support cell membrane. A research team has demonstrated that using trehalose with an enzyme can stimulate nerve fiber growth for getting nerves to reconnect and communicate with the brain."*

In July 2006, I shared the findings at Cornell University from a study reporting that a brain rewired itself in a young man during a 19-year coma.

The Language of LIFE

Glycobiology has opened our understanding to the function of biological sugars that are used in the construction, maintenance and repair of your body's operating system. Indeed, it is the highly functional biological sugars that are responsible for communication among all the cells of your body. This is in stark contrast to simple table sugars that hinder healthy cellular signals.

The study of these essential sugars is Glycobiology (glyco is Greek for sugar). Glycans formed by these special sugars give us life and intelligence. We call them "Smart Sugars." Some 800,000 antenna-like sugar transceivers sugar coat each healthy human cell like fuzz on a peach. These transceivers are constructed from mannose, fucose, galactose, xylose, N-acetylglucosamine, glucose, and variations of other specific Smart Sugars.

Each transceiver is a glycan or glycoprotein. A glycan is a tiny tree-like structure of different sugars linked together. A glycoprotein is made of sugar and protein links. Without an abundance of healthy glycans, the cell cannot live or communicate properly.

Language, Tone, and Volume of Glycoprotein Signals to Modulate Cytokines for Proper Immune Response

The language, tone, and volume of glycoprotein signals hold the key to the future of medical science. They hold the key to the ultimate diagnostic analysis. Understanding these codes will enable us to better see the battlefield of hidden health challenges. As we learn the language, tone, and volume of these signals, we can better develop the strategies for winning the battles. Every cell of the human body is transmitting signals in its cry for help or simply in its request for proper nutrition.

In this posting you will see that scientists are pushing the boundaries and peering into the possibilities for new diagnostic tools. Let us look at the research done here in the US on the IL-8 protein and then look at the work with the IL-8 work done in France for modulating cytokine response via glycoprotein coding on a virus and we gain new understanding of viral infections.

Scientists continue to verify the conclusive and unchallenged importance of the glycoproteins. Our understanding of the language of glycoproteins is not as important today as the cells understanding each other. The cells understand the glycoprotein language, tone and they regulate the volume when there are enough healthy glycoprotein receptor sites to do so.

While waiting on all the coming diagnostic technology, let us invest our time and money eating the nutrients that are the building blocks for the glycoproteins. Let us grow an abundance of glycoprotein receptor sites and we may discover that the coming diagonostic analysis will report good health.

Source and References:
https://www.sciencedaily.com/releases/2008/08/080801074048.htm
https://www.ncbi.nlm.nih.gov/pubmed/16725233

Sugars in Breast Milk Help Nursing Mothers with Multiple Sclerosis

Studies have shown for years that Smart Sugars are beneficial when fed to new born babies. These sugars improve the child's mental and mobility skills for the rest of their lives. These specific sugars are provided by nature in human mothers' breast milk.

But, what about the mother who makes and provides these sugars to their nursing infants?

The Journal of American Medical Association – JAMA/Archives reveal interesting information that we are contemplating in today's Smart Sugar Lesson.

Some of the work reported here was supported by the National Institutes of Health (NIH), National Institute of Neurological Disorders and Stroke Patient-Oriented Research Career Development Award, and a Wadsworth Foundation Young Investigator Award.

The mother also benefits from producing these sugars. Evidence is in showing that women with Multiple Sclerosis have a reduced risk of relapse, EVEN WHEN SHE NURSES THE INFANT FOR ONLY TWO MONTHS. Nursing longer is normally significantly better for both the mother and child.

Multiple sclerosis (MS) is a chronic inflammatory disease of the central nervous system. Royal Sugars that reduce inflamation, improve the immune system, and help MS patients, are proving to be beneficial toward helping many other neurodegenerative diseases. Sugars that modulate the immune system are vital for MS and other autoimmune diseases.

Evidence from the studies showed that the women with MS and healthy women who exclusively breastfed had significantly prolonged lactational amenorrhea [absence of menstruation], which is associated with a decreased risk of relapse in women with MS.

We encourage mothers and soon-to-be-mothers to resist the temptation for convenience of the infant formulas and to go the natural route. Only within the more recent "advance civilization" has humans ignored nature's ways and means of infant feeding.

I have witnessed new born babies receiving significant health benefits from Smart Sugars after the mother repeatedly dampened her little finger, dipped in into the sugars then placed in the baby's mouth.

We have the world's most advance medical culture for treating trauma. However, when it comes to healthcare, we have allowed drugs to replace nutrition, a quick fix to replace prevention, and fast foods to replace good diets. But, wait a minute, what could be better nutrition, better prevention, and faster food than mothers' milk for that precious child.

New findings verify that old findings were right. Our parents, grandparents, and ancestors going back to the beginning of human civilization were giving children the best start in life. No infant formula can hold a candle to the quality and benefits of human mothers' breast milk because of the natural Royal Sugars.

Source and References:

http://sciencedaily.com/releases/2009/06/090608162432.htm

http://www.endowmentmed.org/pdf/SmartLesson34.pdf

Smart Sugars Are Abundant in Mother's Breast Milk

Smart Sugars are abundant in mothers' breast milk and are essential for a healthy start in life. These special sugars orchestrate the construction of every detail of new life. They are the building blocks for prenatal and postnatal development. The nursing mother provides colostrum and milk loaded with Smart Sugar nutrients to supply her baby with a balanced and modulated immune system. Smart Sugars directly improve the immune system, and immunology plays a major role in repairing, recovering and prevention. The quality of the baby's immune system determines the quality of the health and natural mental and motor abilities throughout adult life.

Multiple studies verify that children who receive mothers' milk are smarter and healthier. Harvard University published a paper in 2013 that concludes that children who nurse for twelve months have a four-point IQ advantage over children who nurse for only six months.

Scientists Discover How
To Increase Children's IQ
Smart Sugars can help a mother increase her child's IQ by 4 points

Evidence is in that Smart Sugars in a human breast-fed babies improve the intelligence of the child for many years, perhaps for life.

I have reported on these university studies over the years; but, now several institutions in Massachusetts and Washington state provide us with actual Intelligent Quota (IQ) increase data.

Scientists and researchers in Boston Children's Hospital, Harvard Medical School, and Harvard School of Public Health assessed 1,312 mothers and children. Results showed that the longer mothers exclusively breast-fed their babies, the better those children did at age three on a vocabulary test, and at age seven on an intelligence test.

Journal of the American Medical Association Pediatrics (JAMA Pediatrics) quotes the researchers, *"Our results support a causal relationship of breast-feeding duration with receptive language and verbal and nonverbal intelligence later in life."*

The benefits of the Smart Sugars go beyond mental improvements. According to Dr. Dimitri Christakis of the Seattle Children's Research Institute, breast-feeding also lessens problems with gastroenteritis and ear infections.

Breast feeding cognitive effects are lifelong, Christakis stated, *"It is clear that a vicious cycle can be created wherein lack of breast-feeding begets lower IQ, which begets lower socioeconomic status and thereby decreases the probability of breast-feeding the next generation and so on."* Many women breast-feed their newborns, but only 35% continue after 6 months.

One of the researchers concluded, *"Let's allow our children's cognitive function be the force that tilts the scale, and let's get on with it."* With this statement, he was struggling with the frustration of children forever being not as smart as they could be if only they could receive plenty of mothers' milk for a longer period of time. The Massachusetts researchers discovered that breast-feeding a baby for one year actually increases that child's IQ by about four points.

Pioneers in the field of natural Glycoscience have evidenced the continual benefit of supplementing Smart Sugars for newborns. We have recommended allowing the infant to suck on the tip of the parent's clean finger after it is moistened and coated with these important plant saccharides. Mannose seems to be one of the most, if not the most, influential member in the family of Smart Sugars. It is present in the glycan coating of the surface of human cells even when some of the other sugars are missing. The more abundant the glycans, the healthier the cell. The healthier the cells, the healthier the human body.

The Endowment for Medical Research has two peer-reviewed papers published evidencing improved brain function in adults using plant polysaccharides. We now have scientific evidence of improved brain function of all ages from infant to nearly a century old.

Glycoscience is science's relative new term for the discipline of biology that gives life and intelligence to the human race.

Source and References:

http://www.endowmentmed.org/pdf/SmartLesson100.pdf

Do Smart Sugars Provide LIFE to the Blood?
What exactly are Glycoproteins?

Conflicts in life and health, human and cellular, are resolved only with good communication. When the internal human communication system is faulty, it sustains, compounds, and may even cause the very problem it was designed to inhibit. Human cells in conflict cause toxic infection which is the ultimate cause of most deaths.

Glycoproteins and glycolipids read, transcribe, and process your DNA and RNA, giving instructions for your very life. Smart Sugars joined together with certain proteins are the building blocks for constructing Glycoproteins that coat healthy cells like fuzz on a peach.

Glycoproteins are much more than just the OS of the human body. With only a few decades of glycoprotein research and scientific study behind us, the interest is accelerating because we now know Glycoproteins hold important keys to life itself.

It is the design, the composition and folding of glycoprotein structures that dictate their various functions. The sugar to protein ratio in the total mass of the structures range from less than one percent (1%) to more than eighty percent (80%).

Ongoing research has recently been expanded to determine glycoprotein cluster composition to learn more about their structural function as well as communicational function.

Besides communication, Glycoproteins provide cell to cell adhesion. They are protective agents and lubricants and are also found abundantly in the blood plasma where they serve many more functions.

The superfamily of Smart Sugars are saccharides of different chain lengths. There are some 200 known Smart Sugar compounds constructed with the building blocks of monosaccharides to polysaccharides. These specific Smart Sugars form more complex sugar molecules that can then be linked to polypeptides (chains of one or more amino acids). A long chain of 50 amino acids makes a protein. Glycoproteins are formed when the proteins are linked to the complex sugar molecules.

Scientists knew the Genome Project would be complex. Then they learned that the Glycome Project may be a thousand times more complex and even more exciting because it is getting closer to what determines LIFE and

DEATH. The genes hold the secret to reproduction of LIFE while Smart Sugars determine blood type, provide the OS for the DNA, and bring LIFE or DEATH to the cell.

The function of the Glycoproteins is determined by how these complex Smart Sugars are arranged and bonded together to form the longer chain polysaccharides and how these chains are bonded to the protein. The sugars have two possible linkage formations to their protein partners, either a N-glycosidic bond or an O-glycosidic (N/O) bond. These N/O sugar bonds allow alkaline and acid to be handled differently.

The vast functional diversity of the glycoprotein's roles is determined by the two basic glycosidic structures.   Understanding the N/O bond is a quantum leap in glycoprotein research. Smart Sugars provide not only your blood type but they provide LIFE to your blood.

Source and References:
http://www.endowmentmed.org/pdf/SmartLesson100.pdf

Smart Sugars and Blood

LIFE is in the blood and your blood is unique to you. There are four basic blood types: A, B, AB and O. Each blood type is determined by how precisely the Smart Sugars are arranged on the surface of the cells. Just one sugar differentiates the blood types. That one sugar has the power to determine life or death. If Type A blood is transfused into a Type B individual, the sugar structures on the surface of the immune cells identify that one sugar as different and signals that a foreign agent is in the blood. These Smart Sugar structures instruct the immune cells to destroy all the intruder blood cells which can result in the recipient's death.

However, Type O blood, the universal blood donor, can often be safely transfused to all blood types because all four of its determining sugars are recognized by the defense cells and are accepted. Type AB blood is called the universal blood receiver because it has both the A and B sugar patterns which are recognized and deemed acceptable.

[This simplistic explanation of blood type does not cover the + and − factors that involve an additional protein.]

Blood and Sugar ¤
Your Circulatory System, the Highway of LIFE

The glucose spike is just the tip of the iceberg of the sugar problem. When your sugar is off, your health is off. Sugars determine everything about your body including your blood type. Your LIFE is literally held in the four parts of your blood: red blood cells, white blood cells, platelets, and the plasma in which your life is suspended. Your circulatory system is controlled by sugars. Your OS is Glycoproteins on the surface of your cells.

The highway of LIFE is literally your body's circulatory system made up of a vast network of pipe extending 50,000 to 70,000* miles. Your veins and arteries are the super highways and your capillaries are the back road vessels that take your blood and nutrients to the most remote regions of your body. Some lanes are so narrow that the blood cells must pass single file. The blood passes through your heart twice per cycle which takes about one minute to make the journey through your body.

Healthy bones are vitally important because it is there in the marrow where you manufacture approximately two million (2,000,000) new blood cells EVERY SECOND. That is 120 million per minute, 7.2 billion per hour, nearly 173 billion new blood cells per day. The correct ratio of healthy red blood cells and healthy white blood cells is communicated through the OS via the Glycoproteins. When communication is faulty, too many or not enough red or white blood cells are produced and maintained. Communication is PARAMOUNT.

LIFE is in the blood. The job of your blood is to supply everything your body needs and to emove everything your body does not need. Your blood performs according to its health, the quality of your heart, and how clear is your circulatory system. The health of the blood determines how well you receive oxygen, water, and nutrition throughout your body which in turn determines the health of all your organs. Clean air, clean water, and adequate wholesome nutrition maintains good health. The quality of LIFE is reduced and LIFE shortened when pollutants are put into your body if they are not removed.

In addition to everything else, your circulatory system regulates the temperature of your body. Should you overheat, an air conditioning system is turned on; you perspire and the evaporation cools. Exercise and deep breathing brings more oxygen into the system and to your brain.

The blood's sugar load spikes when high glycemic sugars or foods are consumed. The sugar industry has declared that sugar does not cause diabetes but may cause obesity which causes diabetes. And, high fructose corn syrup (HFCS) compounds the problem while the marketers simply reply, "Sugar is sugar." Bad sugars cause or contribute to many diseases.

In another lesson, I will deal with the different blood types and how just one sugar is the reason you have your blood type. The cutting edge science of GLYCOMICS is here to stay and impact the medical field, all of healthcare, and change the way we live.

*Estimates range from 50,000 to 100,000 miles

Source and References:

http://www.endowmentmed.org/content/view/1160/1/

Blood Mobility

Life is in the blood, nourishing all cells. When red blood cells have a high population of glycans they also have greater flow mobility. Glycans make the cells slippery and able to travel more easily though our ~100,000 miles of blood vessels. This lubricating factor alone improves health. Unrestricted mobility provides a healthier cardiovascular system that can deliver Smart Sugars and other nutrients to the cells. This lubrication is especially needed in the finest of capillaries where blood flow is restricted to the width of a single blood cell.

Tools for Repairing Your Neurons with New Stem Cells - Studies reveal damaged brains and spinal cords benefit from Smart Sugar

Regenerative Strategies of Spinal Cord Injury

Have you ever laid awake at night wondering how embryonic stem cells decide what they want to be when they grow up? Embryonic stem cells have not yet been instructed how to repair or build functional cell structures and organs. No scientist understands exactly how they decide, but we have discovered that mannose and other Smart Sugars help them make the right choices. If they make the wrong choice, it can mean death.

Put on your microscope and let us look at how we can work with stem cells. The neurotrophic factor is vital in the development of stem cells. Neurotrophins deal with the nourishing of embryonic neurons to help them grow up to be well mannered adult cells. The neuropeptides regulate the growth, survival, and deciding factors.

Neurotrophins help design and program the stem cells for the job needed anywhere in the body. Instructions are given for them to migrate to the designated area of the brain or region of the body to begin their work.

Like the rest of your body, stem cells need proper nutrition. With proper exercise you improve blood flow throughout the body with about 25% of the oxygen going to the brain. Rehydration is more much important than most people understand. Very few people drink enough clean water needed to flush out the trash.

Regeneration of neurons is important for everyone if they have neurodegenerative challenges or not. We have learned that we can stimulate stem cell proliferation within the human body with specific sugars. Neural-specific glycosylation of the embryo demonstrates the cell's potential role and interactive influence. As stem cells mature, glycan expressions are ready to direct damage control of tissue.

The neurotrophic factor was included in a recent study dealing with enhancing the neurotrophin-3 (NT-2) bioactivity. The sugar Trehalose was shown to be the most effective additive for stabilizing NT-3 during sonication (sound waves) and lyophilization (freeze drying). Another study conducted in 2001 concerned nerve growth factor in the treatment of neuronal diseases and used Trehalose in the formulation to protect the cells from degradation.

There is a new found hope for those with cognitive impairment and some people are seeing reversal of memory problems. Help arrives in the form of regular exercise combined with a proper diet and Smart Sugars. Each stem cell, and every cell for that matter, have glycan instructions and an operations manual unique for the challenge the human body has right now. The proper care and feeding of the glycans is paramount. The reason for today's health challenges may be that the glycans have not been properly cared for as in days gone by. But, this is a new day filled with new insight.

Neurotrophins containing high-mannose glycosylation are critical to our optimization of mental and motor skills. These molecule building blocks contribute to structure of the neurons and action of the neurotransmitters. Individuals with neurodegenerative challenges, as with Alzheimer's disease, have been shown to have much lower levels of neurotrophins than more normal functioning brains.

The cell's development and function depend on its portfolio of Smart Sugars. We see high-mannose glycans take the lead role in coupling other sugars with proteins to provide actual packages of messages. Scientists were surprised to discover the communication is quite complex, containing detailed blueprints for repair or construction of complete organs. The expressed oligosaccharides on the cell reflect the cell's identity and influence its cell interactions and control of pathogens.

Researchers have learned that specific glycosylation, as in fucosylation or mannosylation, provides the stem cell with the ability to induce glycan expressions that complement the previously identified developmental and innate immune functions of the glycoprotein receptors. Your life depends on Smart Sugars.

Source and References:

http://www.molbiolcell.org/content/16/12/5761.full

http://www.endowmentmed.org/pdf/SmartLesson98.pdf

Cell Regeneration

You are a new person every seven to ten years. Glycobiology has taught us that stem cells orchestrate signaling for cell regeneration. As stem cells mature, glycan expressions are made ready to direct damage control of tissue and complete their designed tasks.

The sugar Trehalose can be used in tissue engineering because it strengthens the cell membrane and assists in proper folding of the proteins. Other Smart Sugars aid in neural regeneration and repair.

The regeneration timeline for different parts of the human body varies depending on the immune system and apoptosis (genetically programmed cell death) for regeneration of various cells and organs. Bone marrow and sinew regenerate more rapidly than the bone. Oxygen, calcium and other minerals availability for bone matrix and cartilage also alter the speed of regeneration.

Red blood cells live for about four months. White blood cells normally live more than a year. Your skin cells live two to three weeks. Colon cells die off after about four days. Sperm cells have a short life span of about three days while brain cells typically last the lifetime of the owner. In the past, it was taught that neurons in the brain are not replaced when they die, but evidence seems to indicate they do. Synapses are literally created almost instantly by new thoughts of a healthy brain. Stem cell regeneration holds many questions. Some researchers say stem cells live for five months to three years. Other reports indicate they may live longer.

Source and References:

http://www.endowmentmed.org/content/view/1325/106/

Brain rewired itself in a coma miracle
Study of man who spent 19 years in 'vegetative state'

In a medical study sure to remind the world of the debate surrounding the forced dehydration death of Terri Schiavo, researchers found the injured brain of a man in a "vegetative state" for 19 years rewired itself, permitting him to renew communication with his loved ones.

The findings by Nicholas Schiff and his colleagues at Weill Medical College at Cornell University suggest the human brain shows far greater potential for recovery and regeneration then ever before suspected.

Source and References:

http://www.endowmentmed.org/content/view/562/106/

Faulty and False Communication

When our cells have an abundance of healthy glycans coating the cellular transceivers, things work more effectively in the body. Simply stated, when we don't, things go awry. *We now know from the study of Glycoscience that every ailment, every disease, all sickness is the result of faulty communication.* Even a split second of non-communication or faulty communication during a baby's nine month gestation period can cause spina bifida deformities.

Faulty signals can render your immune system dysfunctional. It may become weak and ineffective, or confused and attack your own body's cells as an autoimmune disorder. Autoimmune and degenerative diseases involve missing sugars on the cell's surface.

Glycoscience teaches us that neuron transmission is damaged by manmade confusion that tangles communication. Information is often blocked completely or the wires are crossed to give a totally different message than intended. The earlier you start in life to build an excellent neurological transmission system the better.

Common Cause Found For
All Neurodegenerative Disorders

We had over a hundred Alzheimer's and Parkinson sufferers in our Pilot Surveys at The Endowment for Medical Research before we knew there was a common cause. The growing family of neurodegenerative disorders include Alzheimer's, Parkinson's, Huntington's, prion encephalopathies and cystic fibrosis. The commonality is misfolded polypeptide chains which are toxic to the cell. Genetic diseases are linked to the loss of function of certain gene properties.

Toxicity in the cell is a major contributing factor to corruption of the signals the cells receive and transmit via their glycoprotein receptor sites. The question appears to be, *"Did the toxins cause the misfolding of the protein or did the misfolding generate the toxins."* While the answer may be, *"Both"*, one thing is for certain; was the corruption of the signals that caused and compounded the abnormality.

Scientists conclude that glycomics deal with sugars. (Genomics deal with genes and proteomics deal with proteins.) Glycoscience is the science that will change the way we address healthcare. Specific saccharides are required for the cells to be healthy and communicate with distinctive signals. Signal corruption may cause abnormalities that lead to Alzheimer's, Parkinson, and Huntington disease. AIDS or other deadly diseases may be caused by viruses as they are formed by the misfolding of proteins.

List of Known Neurological Disorders that are Caused or Accentuated by Improper Folding of the Proteins

This partial list of neurological dysfunctions will continue to grow as scientists discover new variations of neurological disorders. The symptoms and similarities often confuse the issue and result in wrong diagnoses. Sometimes there are overlaps in names because different doctors or researchers find the same or a similar disease and names it after themselves as first to describe the disease, or they name it after their patient as perhaps the first to be diagnosed.

Proper folding of proteins in individuals with one or more of these dysfunctions may find health benefits by improving the folding of the proteins. Research funding is needed to explore the benefits through Quantum Glycobiology. We have already achieved significant benefits in individuals with many of these some 500 dysfunctions:

Absence of the Septum Pellucidum - Acid Lipase Disease - Acid Maltase Deficiency - Acquired Epileptiform Aphasia - Acute Disseminated Encephalomyelitis - Adie's Pupil - Adie's Syndrome - Adrenoleukodystrophy - Agenesis of the Corpus Callosum - Agnosia - Aicardi Syndrome - Alexander Disease - Alpers' Disease - Alternating Hemiplegia - Alzheimer's - Amyotrophic Lateral Sclerosis - Anencephaly - Aneurysm - Angelman Syndrome - Angiomatosis -Antiphospholipid Syndrome - Aphasia - (or aphemia) - Apraxia - Arachnoid Cysts - Arachnoiditis - Arnold-Chiari Malformation - Arteriovenous Malformation - Asperger - Ataxia - Friedreich's ataxia - Ataxia Telangiectasia - Ataxias and Cerebellar or Spinocerebellar Degeneration - Spinocerebellar ataxia - Atrial Fibrillation and Stroke - Autism - Autonomic Dysfunction - Barth Syndrome - Batten Disease - Becker's Myotonia - Behcet's Disease - Bell's Palsy - Benign Essential Blepharospasm - Benign Focal Amyotrophy - Monomelic amyotrophy - Benign Intracranial Hypertension or benign intracranial hypertension - Bernhardt-Roth Syndrome - Binswanger's Disease - or Subcortical Leukoencephalopathy - Blepharospasm - Bloch-Sulzberger Syndrome - Brachial Plexus Injuries - Bradbury-Eggleston Syndrome - Brain and Spinal Tumors - Brain Aneurysm - Brain Injury - Brown-Sequard Syndrome - Bulbospinal Muscular Atrophy or Kennedy's disease - Cadasil (Cerebral Autosomal Dominant Arteriopathy with Sub-cortical Infarcts and Leukoencephalopathy) - Canavan Disease - Carpal Tunnel Syndrome - Causalgia - Cavernomas - Cavernous Angioma - Central Cord Syndrome - Central Pain Syndrome - Central Pontine Myelinolysis - Cephalic Disorders - Ceramidase Deficiency - Cerebellar Degeneration - Cerebellar Hypoplasia - Cerebral Aneurysm - Cerebral Arteriosclerosis - Cerebral Atrophy - Cerebral Beriberi - Cerebral Gigantism (Sotos syndrome) - Cerebral Hypoxia - Cerebral Palsy - Cerebro-Oculo-Facio-Skeletal Syndrome -Charcot-Marie-Tooth Disease - Chiari Malformation - Chorea - Chronic Inflammatory Demyelinating

Polyneuropathy - Chronic Pain - Coffin Lowry Syndrome - Colpocephaly - Coma and Persistent Vegetative State - Congenital Facial Diplegia (Mobius syndrome) - Congenital Myasthenia - Congenital Myopathy - Corticobasal Degeneration - Cranial Arteritis (Vasculitis) - Craniosynostosis - Creutzfeldt-Jakob Disease - Cumulative Trauma Disorders - Cushing's Syndrome - Cytomegalic Inclusion Body Disease - Dancing Eyes-Dancing Feet Syndrome - Dandy-Walker Syndrome - Dawson Disease - Dementia - Dementia - Multi-Infarct - Dementia - Semantic - Frontotemporal dementia - Dementia - Subcortical - Binswanger's disease - Dementia With Lewy Bodies - Dentate Cerebellar Ataxia (Dyssynergia Cerebellaris Myoclonica) - Dentatorubral Atrophy (Dentatorubral pallidoluysian atrophy) - Developmental Dyspraxia - Devic's Syndrome (Neuromyelitis optica) - Diabetic Neuropathy - Diffuse Sclerosis - Dravet Syndrome - Dysautonomia - Dysgraphia -Dyslexia - Dysphagia - Dyssynergia Cerebellaris Myoclonica - Dystonias - Early Infantile Epileptic Encephalopathy (Ohtahara syndrome) Empty Sella Syndrome - Encephalitis - Encephalitis Lethargica - Encephalopathy - Encephalotrigeminal Angiomatosis - Epilepsy - Erb-Duchenne and Dejerine-Klumpke Palsies - Erb's Palsy - Essential Tremor - Extrapontine Myelinolysis - Fabry Disease - Fahr's Syndrome - Fainting (Syncope) - Familial Dysautonomia (Riley-Day syndrome) - Familial Hemangioma (Cavernous malformation) - Familial Idiopathic Basal Ganglia Calcification - Familial Periodic Paralyzes - Familial Spastic Paralysis (Hereditary spastic paraplegia) - Farber's Disease (- also known as Farber's lipogranulomatosis or ceramidase deficiency) - Febrile Seizures - Fetal Alcohol syndrome - Fibromuscular Dysplasia - Fisher Syndrome - Floppy Infant Syndrome (hypotonia or infantile hypotonia) - Foot Drop - Friedreich's Ataxia - Frontotemporal Dementia - Gangliosidoses -Gaucher's Disease - Gerstmann's Syndrome - Gerstmann-Straussler-Scheinker Disease - Giant Cell Arteritis - Giant Cell Inclusion Disease (cytomegalovirus virus) - Globoid Cell Leukodystrophy (Krabbe disease) - Glossopharyngeal Neuralgia - Glycogen Storage Disease (glycogenosis, dextrinosis) - Guillain-Barre Syndrome - Hallervorden-Spatz Disease - Head Injury - Headache (vascular, muscle contraction (tension), traction, and inflammatory) - Hemicrania Continua - Hemifacial Spasm - Hemiplegia Alterans - Hereditary Neuropathies - Hereditary Spastic Paraplegia - Heredopathia Atactica Polyneuritiformis (Adult Refsum disease) - Herpes Zoster (Shingles) - Herpes Zoster Oticus (Ramsay Hunt Syndrome or

Ramsay Hunt Syndrome type II) - Hirayama Syndrome (Monomelic amyotrophy) - Holmes-Adie syndrome - Holoprosencephaly - HTLV-1 Associated Myelopathy - Hughes Syndrome (Antiphospholipid syndrome) - Huntington's Disease - Hydranencephaly - Hydrocephalus - Hydromyelia - Hypersomnia - Hypertonia - Hypotonia - Hypoxia - Immune-Mediated Encephalomyelitis (Acute disseminated encephalomyelitis) - Inclusion Body Myositis (Sporadic inclusion body myositis) - Incontinentia Pigmenti - Infantile Hypotonia -Infantile Neuroaxonal Dystrophy - Infantile Phytanic Acid Storage Disease - Infantile Refsum Disease - Infantile Spasms - Inflammatory Myopathies - Iniencephaly - Intestinal Lipodystrophy (Whipple's disease) - Intracranial Cysts - Intracranial Hypertension (Idiopathic intracranial hypertension or benign intracranial hypertension or pseudotumor cerebri) - Isaac's Syndrome neuromyotonia or Isaac-Mertens syndrome) - Joubert syndrome (Joubert-Boltshauser syndrome or cerebelloparenchymal disorder IV or familial cerebellar vermis agenesis or cerebello-oculo-renal syndrome - Kearns-Sayre Syndrome - Kennedy's Disease (Kinsbourne syndrome or Opsoclonus myoclonus syndrome) - Kleine-Levin Syndrome - Klippel-Feil Syndrome - Klippel-Trenaunay Syndrome - Kluver-Bucy Syndrome - Korsakoff's Amnesic Syndrome (Korsakoff's psychosis or amnesic-confabulatory syndrome) - Krabbe Disease (globoid cell leukodystrophy or galactosylceramide lipidosis) - Kugelberg-Welander Disease (Spinal Muscular Atrophy Types I, II, and III) - Kuru -Lambert-Eaton Myasthenic Syndrome - Landau-Kleffner Syndrome - Lateral Medullary Syndrome (Wallenberg's syndrome or posterior inferior cerebellar artery syndrome) - Learning Disabilities - Leigh's Disease (Subacute Necrotizing Encephalomyelopathy) - Lennox-Gastaut Syndrome - Lesch-Nyhan Syndrome (Nyhan's syndrome) - Leukodystrophy - Levine (Critchley Syndrome) - Lewy Body Dementia - Lipid Storage Diseases (lipidoses) - Lipoid Proteinosis - Lissencephaly - Locked-In Syndrome - Lou Gehrig's Disease (ALS or Amyotrophic lateral sclerosis) - Lupus (Neurological Sequelae or lupus erythematosus) - Lyme Disease - Machado-Joseph Disease (spinocerebellar ataxia) - Macrencephaly - Melkersson-Rosenthal Syndrome - Meningitis - Menkes Disease - Meralgia Paresthetica - Metachromatic Leukodystrophy (Arylsulfatase A deficiency) - Microcephaly - Migraine -Miller Fisher Syndrome - Mini-Strokes (TIA - transient ischemic attack) - Mitochondrial Myopathies - Motor Neuron Diseases - Moyamoya Disease - Mucolipidoses - Mucopolysaccharidoses - Multiple System Atrophy - Muscular Dystrophy - Myasthenia Gravis -

Myoclonus - Myopathy - Myotonia -Narcolepsy - Neuroacanthocytosis - Neurodegeneration with Brain Iron Accumulation - Neurofibromatosis - Neurofibromatosis 1 (Recklinghausen's Disease) - Neuroleptic Malignant Syndrome - Neurological Complications of AIDS - Neurological Complications Of Lyme Disease - Neurological Consequences of Cytomegalovirus Infection - Neurological Manifestations of Pompe Disease - Neurological Sequelae Of Lupus - Neuromyelitis Optica or Devic's disease - Neuromyotonia (Isaacs' Syndrome) - Neuronal Ceroid Lipofuscinosis (Batten Disease) - Neuronal Migration Disorders - Neuropathy-Hereditary - Neurosarcoidosis - Neurotoxicity - Nevus Cavernosus (cavernous angioma) - Niemann-Pick Disease - Normal Pressure Hydrocephalus - Occipital Neuralgia - Occult Spinal Dysraphism Sequence (Tethered spinal cord syndrome) - Ohtahara Syndrome - Olivopontocerebellar Atrophy - Opsoclonus Myoclonus - Orthostatic Hypotension (postural hypotension or orthostatic reflect or orthostatic intolerance or colloquially) - O'Sullivan-McLeod Syndrome (Monomelic amyotrophy) - Overuse Syndrome (Carpal Tunnel Syndrome) - Pantothenate Kinase-Associated Neurodegeneration (Hallervorden-Spatz syndrome) - Paraneoplastic Syndromes - Paresthesia - Parkinson's Disease - Paroxysmal Choreoathetosis - Paroxysmal Hemicrania - Parry-Romberg - Pelizaeus-Merzbacher Disease - Perineural Cysts - Periodic Paralyzes (Familial periodic paralyzes) - Peripheral Neuropathy - Periventricular Leukomalacia - Pervasive Developmental Disorders - Pinched Nerve - Piriformis Syndrome - Pompe Disease - Porencephaly - Postherpetic Neuralgia - Postinfectious Encephalomyelitis (Acute disseminated encephalomyelitis) - Post-Polio Syndrome - Post Traumatic Stress ~~Disorder~~ - (PTS~~D~~) - Postural Hypotension (Orthostatic hypotension) - Postural Orthostatic Tachyardia Syndrome - Primary Lateral Sclerosis - Prion Diseases (Transmissible spongiform encephalopathies) - Progressive Multifocal Leukoencephalopathy - Progressive Sclerosing Poliodystrophy (Alpers' disease) - Progressive Supranuclear Palsy - Prosopagnosia - Pseudotumor Cerebri - Ramsay Hunt Syndrome I - Ramsay Hunt Syndrome II - Rasmussen's Encephalitis - Reflex Sympathetic Dystrophy Syndrome - Refsum Disease (Adult Refsum disease) - Refsum Disease - Repetitive Motion Disorders - Repetitive Stress Injuries (cumulative trauma disorder) - Restless Legs Syndrome (Wittmaack-Ekbom's syndrome or Nocturnal myoclonus) - Retrovirus-Associated Myelopathy (Tropical Spastic Paraparesis) - Rett Syndrome - Reye's Syndrome - Rheumatic Encephalitis

(Sydenham chorea) - Riley-Day Syndrome - Saint Vitus Dance (Sydenham chorea) - Sandhoff Disease - Schizencephaly - Septo-Optic Dysplasia - Shaken Baby Syndrome -Shingles (herpes zoster) - Shy-Drager Syndrome - Sjogren's Syndrome - Sleep Apnea - Sleeping Sickness - Sotos Syndrome - Spasticity - Lou Gehrig's disease (ALS or Amyotrophic lateral sclerosis and phenylketonuria) - Spinal Cord Infarction - Spinal Cord Injury - Spinal Cord Tumors (brain and spinal cord tumors) - Spinocerebellar Atrophy - Spinocerebellar Degeneration - Stiff-Person Syndrome - Striatonigral Degeneration - Stroke (cerebral vascular accident or CVA) - Sturge-Weber Syndrome - SUNCT Headache (Short-lasting, Unilateral, Neuralgiform headache attacks with Conjunctival injection and Tearing) - Syncope - Syphilitic Spinal Sclerosis (Tabes dorsalis or Syringomyelia) - Tardive Dyskinesia - Tarlov Cysts - Tay-Sachs Disease (GM2 gangliosidosis Hexosaminidase or Sphingolipidosis deficiency) - Temporal Arteritis (giant cell arteritis) - Tethered Spinal Cord Syndrome - Thomsen's Myotonia - Thoracic Outlet Syndrome - Thyrotoxic Myopathy - Tic Douloureux (Trigeminal neuralgia - Todd's Paralysis (postictal paresis/paralysis "after seizure") - Tourette Syndrome - Transient Ischemic Attack - Transmissible Spongiform Encephalopathies (prion diseases) - Transverse Myelitis - Traumatic Brain Injury (intracranial injury or simply head injury) Tremor - Trigeminal Neuralgia (Tic Douloureux or prosopalgia) - Tropical Spastic Paraparesis - Troyer Syndrome - Tuberous Sclerosis (tuberous sclerosis complex) - Vasculitis (includes Temporal Arteritis) - Von Economo's Disease (Encephalitis lethargica) - Von Hippel-Lindau Disease - Von Recklinghausen's Disease (Neurofibromatosis 1) - Wallenberg's Syndrome (Lateral medullary syndrome or posterior inferior cerebellar artery syndrome) - Werdnig-Hoffman Disease (Infantile spinal muscular atrophy or spinal muscular atrophy type 1 or "spinal muscular atrophy type I") - Wernicke-Korsakoff Syndrome or Wernicke's encephalopathy - West Syndrome (infantile spasms) - Whiplash - Whipple's Disease - Williams Syndrome (Williams-Beuren syndrome) - Wilson's Disease - Wolman's Disease (Wolman's syndrome or acid lipase deficiency) - X-Linked Spinal and Bulbar Muscular Atrophy (Kennedy disease) - Zellweger Syndrome.

Your Brain Is Hardwired For Truth

False Signals Cause Chaos

False signals, sooner or later, develop chaos. Lack of any communication is more trust worthy than miscommunication. False signals make it so you do not know where you are going and that is where you are likely to end up. Lack of communication simply stops all progress.

Your neurons are HARD WIRED for Truth, and Truth is what holds all things together. A few years ago I wrote these words: *Total Truth gives no false signals. The flow of even the slightest false witness gives the wrong signal and initiates the flow of wrong energy and matter. Opinions do not count as Truth. Because nothing is as it appears, what you perceive as reality is in fact, at least in part, an illusion. Untruth is an illusion paralleled with deception.*

The main *function* between components and *systems* is to flow Truth (no false signals), energy, and matter needed by the other components and systems.

The mind is a wonderful thing to waste not. When your brain believes wrong is right, it will sincerely make the wrong choice. I call that negative faith operating on false data.

A hypochondriac may develop an illness in an otherwise healthy body. The brain obeys the <u>constant signals</u> of welcoming illness because it becomes convinced that the <u>signal</u> is Truth. Not only is the hypochondriac affected by this hidden lie, but others as well, including the family, friends, and community. Untruth affects everyone it comes in contact with.

Researchers in brain function at the California Institute of Technology have discovered the region of the brain where struggles with emotion takes place. This published university research helps substantiate that, indeed, Your neurons are HARD WIRED for Truth. The researchers used the fairness, struggles with emotion to find equitable solutions.   They pinpointed the region of the brain where this concept of fairness is processed, the insular cortex, or insula, which is also the seat of emotional reactions.

"The fact that the brain has such a robust response to unfairness suggests that sensing unfairness is a basic evolved capacity," notes Steven Quartz, an associate professor of philosophy at Caltech and author of the study.

We have developed a pathway to improve brain function with Smart Sugars that are the building blocks for the Operating System (OS) of the brain and every cell of your body. Communication between cells is the responsibility of the Smart Sugars. However, the choice of morality, the choice of Truth is left up to the individual. Truth is hardwired into the brain.

When you go against Truth, your whole body knows and responds with a compounding stress level. Stress causes aging and the need to improve the immune system. Smart Sugars improve immunity and reduce stress.

Source and References:

Smart Sugars Lesson #77 http://www.endowmentmed.org/pdf/SmartLesson77

Chapter Four

A Look at a Tiny Virus

*"Our only real competitors
for dominion of the planet
remain the viruses."*
Nobel laureate, Dr. Joshua Lederberg

Should you think that little tiny SYSTEMS are not important, listen to the words of the Nobel laureate, Dr. Joshua Lederberg, "*Our only real competitors for dominion of the planet remains the viruses.*"

A single virus is a tiny evil commando that doesn't eat, secrete, or propel itself. It is unable to reproduce without the aid of another living cell. The virus follows its pre-programmed instructions to reprogram the cells of another organism making that organism the host.

By reprogramming the host cell the virus causes that cell to become a traitor directing it to cease its DESIGNED FUNCTION. and instead to replicate the invader producing clones of the virus.

"*The virus then seizes key positions in the host's body and spreads to other hosts-in-waiting at the first opportunity.*

"*Some viruses attack and disable their victims with cruel speed. ... Other viruses take years to harm their hosts. AIDS can incubate for up to a decade, allowing the deadly agent plenty of time to pass to new hosts before its ill-effects become apparent. Others* [viruses], *such as herpes simplex, co-exists so well we're often unaware of their presence.*"

It has been said that the flu virus has a thousand lives. We can catch the flu many times over because of its prodigious capability to genetically change. The virus contains substances called antigens. Each viruses' antigens have tiny spots on their surfaces that fit onto a certain section of the antibody, similar to a key in a lock. Upon contact of an antibody with the virus, a command signal is given and the antigen is disabled resulting in the disappearance of the flu symptoms.

Viruses mutate quickly changing their combination or signals. An ever so slight mutation of the antigens is all that is necessary to negate all the antibodies that have been resident for years. This enables the virus to infect you all over again and again and again. A new antibody must be produced to go after the newly DESIGNED invaders.

Morse and Brown conclude that "*if we don't take steps to monitor and contain their* [viruses'] *continual thrusts, one of their sorties could one day erupt into a global pandemic."* End of quote from my earlier writings.

Cognizant and physical responses from many causes including viruses have been documented to be improved when the science of Glycomics is integrated into the equation.

What is The Virus?

Early on in my studies, I was fascinated by a significant example of false communication that causes so much havoc in the human body: the virus.

The virus is a key counterfeiter. A single virus is a tiny evil commando that appears dead. It does not eat, secrete, or propel itself. It is unable to reproduce without the aid of a living cell.

DNA and RNA viruses are intracellular parasites that implement their evil plans by communicating false information to the cell. The message is, *"Don't reproduce yourself; reproduce me, here is my code."*

Viruses seize key positions on the surface of cells. Some viruses attack and disable their victims with cruel speed, while other viruses take years to harm their host. A virus, as in guerrilla warfare, lies in wait for a more opportune time to attack when your immune defenses are lowered.

Viruses and Smart Sugars

Viruses are the greatest example of evil personified. A virus is worse than a parasite which simply feeds on and lives off of another life. A virus is powerless on its own and like a parasite, attaches itself to another life form. The virus can speak cell language. Unable to reproduce on its own, the virus signals this message to the host cell, *"Don't reproduce yourself. Reproduce Me! Here is my DNA. Accept it as your own."*

The targeted host cell can accept the DNA or RNA of the virus when its defenses are down. It loses its ability to reproduce itself and reproduces a copy of the virus. Reprogramming the DNA of another cell is the only way that a virus can propagate. The deceptive virus is at war with us and scientists agree that it is the one single greatest threat for annihilation of the human race.

When the human host cell is weak it has no choice but to heed the voice of the enemy. When the human host cell is strong, healthy, and supported with a viable immune system it automatically and instinctively rejects the virus. The alarmed cell makes at least two immediate responses (cell calls if you will). 1) *"Don't even think about docking your deceiving viral vessel in this harbor. My receptor sites are loaded and there is no room for you."* 2) By cell-to-cell communication the endangered cell sends an alert signal to summon the mother of all big eaters, the macrophage.

The macrophage (Greek for big eater) is a powerful warrior against toxins and infections except in bodies with poor immune systems they are hard of hearing and less active. The macrophage is a specific type of white blood cell that disables and ingests foreign invaders of the body. A macrophage is usually immobile and loosely connected to blood vessel walls. They are both a nonspecific defense system for a good immune system and specific defense when needed for a specified purpose, like this deadly virus.

The macrophage is battle ready and silently awaiting the command. The macrophage is awakened by the cry of a healthy cell in trouble. With an amazing complex and harmonious coordination, the macrophage recognizes, attacks, and removes the virus and other invading particles. When needed, the macrophage marches in lock-step with another white blood cell, the helper T-cell, to provide protection to the body.

When the cell-to-cell communication is operating properly, the macrophage may come alone or summon an army to the battle. One macrophage can battle and devour 100 bacteria. We may not yet understand all the troops needs for viral battles but we have seen some amazing battles won by increasing the amount of Smart Sugars in the human body.

A virus can dock on a cell surface if the glycoprotein receptor sites are sparse. The cell is healthy when the Glycoproteins cover the cell like thick fuzz on a peach. Specific Smart Sugars are not only the building blocks for a good immune system, they construct the Operating System of the body for all communication. That is really important when you need a macrophage.

Source and References:

http://www.endowmentmed.org/pdf/SmartLesson71.pdf

The Good NEWS

The good news is that understanding and then implementing what Glycoscience is teaching us,will give us better cellular communication and therefore improved health and quality of life. To increase the quality and quantity of the glycans on our cells is called glycosylation.

The structure/function of glycan/glycoprotein receptors provide for proper folding of these glycoforms. Proper folding provides the human body with good neurological function for mental and motor skills. Misfolding is the cause for neurological dysfunction. Research shows that the sugar Trehalose is beneficial in proper folding of proteins. The secret is found in how best to safely implement the folding.

Monitoring Glycosylation

Glycoscience provides the ultimate pathway to extend and move biomarkers of life and health.

Data gathering for the human glycome and genome during the past decade surpassed that of all previous generations. Man is, indeed, amassing greater knowledge than anytime in history. Universities worldwide are making astounding glycomic discoveries that will alter medical direction.

The past decade of glycomics started as a continuation of the previous decade of ridicule and disbelief of any possible health benefits from plant polysaachrides taken orally. Papers were published about how glycosylation did not result from the consumption of Smart Sugars.

Those papers were refuted by a team of researchers in England lead by Dr. John Axford when a paper was published in the European Journal of Clinical Nutrition dealing with proven glycosylation of human cells caused by plant-derived polysaccharides. The in-vitro and in-vivo studies suggested that the saccharide biopolymers can have bifidogenic and/or immunomodulatory effect that impact cellular glycosylation.

By the close of 2012 leading U.S. Government agencies had assembled a stellar group of glycoscientists who formed a committee to develop the roadmap for the future of glycomics. The project title was "Transforming Glycoscience". Glycosylation is now recognized paramount to medical research by NIH, FDA, National Science Foundation (NSF), the National Academy of Sciences, and the National Research Council.

It is easier to gather data than ever before because of advanced technologies, but data in a vacuum isn't all that useful. It is reported that Steve Jobs spend $100,000 to gather his personal gene data. In this current decade, we will learn what to do with some of the data. The speed of gathering data is faster than ever before. And the storage cost has moved from $1 million/Tb to less than $50 today. Speed of processing has moved from MHz to Pflops which takes computer mining to a whole new level.

The genome is believed to contain only 30% of the health biomarkers while the glycome may contain the other 70%. Much research is needed and this fact will forever change medical practice.

Universities are pursuing glycomic research at an all time high and disseminating their new found knowledge. As new discoveries of the glycans emerge we will learn better how they interact with antibodies, proteins, viruses, bacteria and how they relate to human health. Glycoscience holds the key to help us define and understand the molecular qualities of biological interactions.

The Endowment for Medical Research for the past decade has collaborated with universities and research labs in [over a dozen] countries. We are postured to advance this collaboration by helping develop a new standard in Glycoscience diagnostics with a unified platform of various technologies that provide verification of location and movement of the biomarkers of aging and health with the ability to extend those biomarkers.

Source and References:

http://www.endowmentmed.org/content/view/1310/1/

Improving Glycosylation

Optimal glycosylation provides excellent communication which can prevent harmful bacteria and viruses from having a docking station on the cell. Furthermore, identification of the foreign foe is transmitted to the immune cells which attack, disable and carry them out of the body as trash. In addition, instructions are given to produce specific stem cells to protect, maintain and repair specific organs. We have discovered that integrating natural specific sugar supplementation into daily consumption of food will increase glycosylation of cells.

Doctors of Tomorrow Will Focus No Longer on *"disease - treat - cure"*

Physicians will rely on Glycoscience Diagnostics

We can take the focus off *"disease - treat - cure"* and simply discover the best pathway to improve our immune and hormonal systems with Smart Sugars to improve cell communication.

The doctor of the future will have access to the state-of-the-art Glycoscience Diagnostics Centre which will count, evaluate, and monitor some 800,000 glycans / glycoproteins per healthy cell. With a drop of blood, tomorrow's doctor will enable you to know what your cells think before they act.

Fewer glycans on the cell make for a more unhealthy cell. Evaluating glycans lets us know how well the cell was glycosylated. Poor glycosylation makes for a poor immune system that permits harmful bacteria and viruses to take up residence and allows corrupted cells to proliferate.

Glycosylation of cells to produce Glycans and Glycoproteins will forever change healthcare. Tomorrow's doctor will accept Glycoscience and understand that glycans give LIFE to the cell. Glycans sugar coat cells like fuzz on a peach and contain packages of information for processing your DNA to build and maintain proper function of cells and organs. These glycan/glycoprotein antenna determine future propensities for all mental and motor skills.

Glycoscience diagnostics can detect your health years in advance based on how well your cells glycosylate. Glycosylation was deemed impossible until recently. Colleagues have glycosylated human cells, monitored and published papers evidencing improved glycans/glycoproteins with Smart Sugars. My friends, during decades of disbelief and ridicule, heard words similar to what other great men endured.

Never Ever Say, "It Cannot Be Done."

Enjoy this bit of humor about the impossible:

"There is no reason anyone would want a computer in their home."
- Ken Olson, president, chairman and founder of Digital Equipment Corp., 1977

"I think there is a world market for maybe five computers."
- Thomas Watson, chairman of IBM, 1943

"I don't know what use any one could find for a machine that would make copies of documents. It certainly couldn't be a feasible business by itself."
- the head of IBM, refusing to back the idea, forcing the inventor to found Xerox.

"This 'telephone' has too many shortcomings to be seriously considered as a means of communication. The device is inherently of no value to us."
- Western Union internal memo, 1876.

"The wireless music box has no imaginable commercial value. Who would pay for a message sent to nobody in particular?"
- David Sarnoff's associates in response to his urgings for investment in the radio in the 1920s.

"Airplanes are interesting toys but of no military value"
- Marechal Ferdinand Foch, Professor of Strategy, Ecole Superieure de Guerre, France.

"..I can assure you that data processing is a fad that won't last out the year."
- The editor in charge of business books for Prentice Hall, 1957

We have 20/20 hindsight on what could not be but soon was. Talking about 20/20 reminds me of a lady in our studies who was blind. She regained her eyesight and became, to our knowledge, the first blind person in Canadian history to have a drivers license. She regained her vision so that she could drive long distances even into the United States and back. We have had others who were color blind and began seeing in color again. Many people have had floaters disappear which had partially blocked their vision. One individual had floaters so badly that at times he could not drive. He would pull over to the side of the road hoping they would dissipate for awhile so he could drive home. For many years, I personally had a mild case of floaters and they have disappeared. Proper communication makes everything happen.

Source, References and Glossary:
[1]Glycosylat (e) (ed) (ion): process for bonding specific sugars to other sugars and/or proteins to form glycans or glycoproteins; [2]Glycans are linked sugars; [3]Glycoproteins are linked sugars and proteins; www.PubMed.gov Axford JS Glycosylation papers

* The reporting of the historic quotations are subject to verification.

http://www.glycosciencenews.com/pdf/Lesson9.pdf

Glycosylation, Once Scoffed - Now Proven

The food supply of earlier generations naturally contained enough of the Smart Sugars that our bodies could manufacture the important sugars that were missing. Sadly, the farming methods of today, depletion of the soil, green harvesting of fruits and vegetables, and over processing food, have resulted in food sources with little nutrition of earlier times. Fewer Smart Sugars in one's diet leaves missing glycans or poor quality glycans. The concept that ingesting sugars from food has a role in cell communication, was once considered impossible. Sugars were once believed to provide energy only. As recently as the 1990s, the reality that health benefits could be obtained from consuming Smart Sugars was rejected by some scientists since no controlled clinical trials had been conducted. Health benefits of certain sugars have been confirmed in history for thousands of years without knowing they were Smart Sugars.

Quality and quantity of Smart Sugars in the blood can be evaluated.

Major Find in 2011

In 2011, Dr. John Axford, past president of the Royal Society of Medicine, conducted an open label study to evaluate the safety and effects of ingesting certain Smart Sugars from plants, i.e., polysaccharides. The work of Dr. Axford and his team included in vitro and in vivo studies which suggest that certain saccharides have immunomodulatory effects and impact cellular glycosylation. Oral ingestion caused no adverse events and a significant overall shift toward increased sialyation*. Scientists have proved beyond a doubt, that these specific sugars are critical to life and health.

* sialyation *is not to be confused with sylation. Sialyation has to do with sialic acid, a generic term for a derivative of neuraminic acid, a monosaccharide. This Smart Sugar is commonly called N-acetylneuraminic acid and is found in glycoproteins. There is significant concentration of sialic acid in the human brain where it plays a role in neural transmission through the synapsis.*

sylation *has to do with the bonding of molecules. When the word "glyco" is placed in front of "sylation", it means to bond a sugar, i.e. glycosylation. When a specific sugar is bonded, the name of that sugar is placed in front of "sylation." To sylate mannose is mannosylation. To sylate fucose is called fucosylation.*

Glycoscience IS The Road Map for the Future

The top scientific governmental body in Washington, DC, the *National Academy of Sciences* (NAS), is made up of Nobel Prize winners or those nominated by Nobel Prize winners. This distinguished community appointed a panel to publish the 200 page report ***Transforming Glycoscience - A Road Map for the Future***. Here, they went on record in 2012 stating that: "*Glycans impact the structure/function of every living cell in humans, animals, and plants.*" The Academy expanded on the importance of the sugars saying: "*Glycans play roles in almost every biological process and are involved in every major disease*" and "*Elimination of any single class of glycans from an organism results in death.*"

To bring Glycoscience from the recently little known into the mainstream, *Transforming Glycoscience* recommends that all university and high school science departments teach Glycoscience.

The National Academies - NAS, National Academy of Engineering, Institute of Medicine, and National Research Council - consider this science so important that their 10-year goal includes, "*integrating Glycoscience into relevant disciplines in high school, undergraduate and graduate education, and developing curricula and standardized testing for science competency which would increase public as well as professional awareness.*"

The Future

Glycoscience's disruptive technology will forever change our medical system. The future of medicine will include cell regeneration, neurodegenerative repair, development and proliferation of stem cells, and tissue regeneration.

Traditional vs. Functional Medicine

Pharmaceutical companies realize there are big profits to be made utilizing the science of Glycobiology to develop new drugs. They are spending billions of dollars to synthesize the sugars to add to the drugs, believing the drugs will work better.

Advancing diagnostics of glycans will enable scientists to better understand the composition of Smart Sugars and proteins.

In the future, in the traditional mode, most medical professionals will be educated by the drug companies on why they should be prescribing these drugs for their patients.

Functional medicine is the medical practice or treatments that focus on optimal function of the body and its organs, treating the whole system, not just symptoms, usually involving natural approaches.

The GLYCOSCIENCE INSTITUTE foresees Functional Medical physicians will use advanced Glycoscience Diagnostics to evaluate a patient's glycans that forecast what the patient's health will be years in advance. These diagnostics will guide clinics to understand what Smart Sugars are needed.

The GLYCOSCIENCE INSTITUTE teaches that Glycobiology helps people of all ages be healthier by improving the quality of the body's cellular communication system by naturally ncreasing the number of glycans.

The new era of medical exploration of the red planet reveals just how safe it can be when you obey the natural laws. Doctors and patients are learning about and advancing the power of Smart Sugars. Some scientists believe we can have an extended stay on the planet and be in good health for well over 100 years.

Glycoscience pioneers are making "proving ground" discoveries and designing advanced clinics to sustain life beyond normal expectancy and pave the way for future missions. The doctors and scientists of tomorrow will do what has never been done and go where no man has gone before.

We learn from what we envision.

Innovative partnerships of doctors, businessmen, and scientists will blaze a trail for the people to follow. These trail blazers will achieve a satisfaction that few ever have... that of helping the human race know the possibilities of health.

Our teams are making it happen and many people will become a part of the team of their choice. Possibilities will be revealed to all who seek more knowledge. Experts from around the world are collaborating in disciplines of Glycoscience that the world knows little or nothing about.

The GLYCOSCIENCE INSTITUTE was designed to educate and partner with all those who are interested in going to another level of awareness and application. Everyone, regardless of their status or lot in life can benefit from the knowledge of Glycoscience.

We offer classes and private consultation in various disciplines of Glycoscience that will benefit every healthcare professional. Our desire is to better equip and empower doctors to be the best in their field. This is an exciting time to learn about the meticulous work your instructors have achieved in this technology and how Glycoscience will change the world.

Every medical student and pre-med student can benefit from classes at the GLYCOSCIENCE INSTITUTE because it will educate them in what we have learned over two decades and put into practice the knowledge that will help many. The student will learn from authorities in Glycoscience about the trends in healthcare and the future of medicine in detail that you never new was available. One of the biggest paradigm shifts is in its early stage. Those who have the knowledge and anticipate these changes will be better equipped to help their patients and the next generation. The student will gain authority to proceed in the many disciplines that are forging into mainstream medicine. Is there a disease, is there an ailment, that cannot be addressed with enhanced immunology? Is there a person on planet earth that cannot benefit from having a better understanding of Glycoscience?

Every person, sick or well, can benefit from these classes. We want to partner with individuals willing to learn and have the foundational belief of the Father of Medicine, Hippocrates, who said, *"First, do no harm."* Hippocrates believed that from conception to death that no life should be harmed. The Hippocratic Oath is not followed very well today from when he said, *"Let food be thy medicine and medicine be thy food."*

Report: Ongoing Research for Improving the Communication Receptor Sites on the Neurons:

Neurotransmitters are chemicals that help neurons communicate. As I have written throughout the book, glycosylation of the cells improves the neurotransmitters' ability to communicate more clearly and have amplified signals.

When various sugars are available in the body, the compounds or compositions may be useful as tissue protectants including neuroprotectants and cardioprotectants.

Cannabinoid receptors are transported by glycosylated proteins (glycoproteins) involved in transmitting and receiving data involved in physiological processes that include appetite, pain, pleasure, mood, and memory.

There has been much orchestrated confusion about hemp/marijuana cannabidiol (CBD) and tetrahydrocannabinol (THC). I am not a proponent of smoke or any carcinogen pumped into your lungs.

Hemp seed oil (CBD) is not psychoactive as is THC. CBD is antioxidant and neuroprotectant. The molecule appears the same but the bonding is different. The confusion is that in the laboratory two molecules appear to be identical but clinically they are worlds apart in function. We have found that a slight degree of difference in the bond of two atoms. In sugars, the bond provides a drastic difference in functionality. I have written much about this with the sugar Trehalose. While this may not be immediately visible to the eye, sometimes it is. Carbon is carbon but it can appear as coal or diamond.

Two major potential problems appears to be the legality and purity of the oil. Research will prove CBD to be rich in health benefits but a landmine of possible risks amplified by Big Pharma.

In the human body every atom, every molecule, in fact everything functions in collaboration with the Smart Sugars. The function of cannabinoid receptors transported by glycosylated proteins in the brain is determined by the purity of all the molecules. The tipping point is brilliance or madness.

The genome is believed to contain only 30% of the health biomarkers while the glycome may contain the other 70%.

Much research is needed and this fact will forever change medical practice for the better.

Chapter Five

Halt the Death Process
for the Critically Ill
**An integrated procedure that may allow more
time to recover from Death's Tipping Point**

"Halt the Death Process" is an attempt to temporally stop the death process. This is to allow the body to begin the healing process. Some efforts succeed... most fail. Doctors in charge are sometimes in disbelief when the patient makes an "impossible" recovery after feeding them specific toxin free Smart Sugars.

Dying patients provides data that helps us better understand how to halt the death process. Defibrillators are used to restart the heart. When other organs fail drastic measures are also required. We have case studies of patients receiving sugar nutrients that sparked new life. Cases range in age from newborn to very elderly.

Scientists have discovered that certain biological carbohydrates impart energy and intelligence to cells. Universities in several countries are studying how these functional carbohydrates improve neuron function. We have evidence that specific sugars help proliferate stem cell production in the human body. Even diabetics can benefit.

At the GLYCOSCIENCE INSTITUTE in Houston, medical professionals and the general public learn not how to treat or cure any disease. Rather, they learn how to optimize the patient's immune and endocrine systems through glycosylation of specific sensors on the surface of cells. Glycosylation (to add glycans and glycoproteins to the cell surface) is accomplished with specific monosaccharides, disaccharides, and polysaccharides. These food nutrients are taken orally, or for the more critically ill are provided through a feeding tube under doctor supervision. In a special report, I explain how I personally received approval from teams of doctors in major medical institutions in Texas for "dying" patients to halt the death process from reaching the tipping point.

The Secret – Make Smart Sugars Abundant in the Dying Patient in an Attempt to Halt the Death Process – Sometimes it Works. With Research, we will make it happen more often.

Certain Smart Sugars sustain life by keeping cells alive and protected. When Smart Sugars are abundant on the cell surface, no virus or harmful bacteria can penetrate the cell membrane. This is, in part, because the receptor sites are occupied and there are no docking sites available for the intruder.

In a healthy person abundant Smart Sugars make it difficult to even get the flu. Studies show that certain sugars strengthen cell membrane, amplify cell signals, and lubricate the blood cells and capillary walls to improve blood flow for optimal cell nourishment.

How Super Smart Sensors Work

Scientists long to solve the mystery of cell signals. In 1999, Günter Blobel, of the Rockefeller University received the Nobel Prize in Physiology or Medicine for "*the discovery that proteins have intrinsic signals that govern their transport and localisation in the cell*". The term proteomics was coined in 1997, Sugars were still considered primary for energy and were not properly credited for generating cell signals. The significance of Smart Sugars with the proteins was not understood. Now, we are beginning to understand how glycans generate signals without the proteins. It is the sugars within the glycoproteins that generate the signals.

Cell transponders and transceivers function to (1) generate signals, (2) receive signals, (3) relay signals, and (4) transmit signals that contain new data as it is discovered.

Life is in the blood. The mission of the multi-functional sensors on cells is to determine environmental status and provide digital and analog data feedback. Some 800,000 sensors per cell continually process dynamically changing complex information. This data creates serial packets of commands to cleanse an area or organ.

How do the untold number of sensors actually work? As I was pondering my own question, I recalled the time when I was a very small boy with a simple radio headset and crystal, I learned how to change the frequencies to listen to different radio stations. My father told to me the story of a man who build a crystal fireplace in his home. People were terrified believing the house was haunted. The reality was that when the fire changed the temperature of the crystals, the fireplace picked up the strongest radio station in the area. The design of the fireplace served as a radio speaker. No wonder people were terrified.

Glycoscience is based in highly functional sugar molecules that are so fine that several million are on the surface of every healthy cell. Think of these millions of various functional sugars linked together to form the glycan or glycoprotein antennae. My theorem, is that the glycans on the cell are not one of the three common states of matter as solid, liquid, or gas. Rather, the glycans, as they appear and function on the cells, are liquid crystal. They are always active, always flowing, having no positional or orientational order.

The liquid crystal phase of matter is between the solid and the liquid phase. While the glycan liquid crystals do not has a distinctive positional order, they possess some orientational order. Perhaps the glycan's orientational order is amplified in the blood by the parabolic shape of the red blood cells. Think of millions of scanning parabolic scopes coursing through your blood stream gathering, processing, communicating with other cells, and transmitting the data gathered only a split second ago.

Liquid crystals act more like liquid than solid and can be verified by the amount of energy needed for heat transfer. A very weak electric field is needed to accomplish all of their tasks. Research is needed on glycan liquid crystals to determine their capabilities beyond processing data and communication. The behavior of the glycans may be determined by many factors including (as I mention in the our Quantum Glycoscience section) variant thermal conditions, light of various spectrums, rate of radioactive decay, direction of rotation, speed of spin, angle of molecular bonds, strength of molecular bond, gravity, electrical discharge transfer of energy, ions, magnetism, photons, radiation, and other unknown influences.

Obvious much research is needed in the area of glycans as liquid crystals and Quantum Glycoscience. This developing discipline of Glycoscience is the new frontier of medicine and healthcare.

The Smart Sugars are building blocks for nano computing platforms where control is up close to resolve local problems and make repairs. Stem cells are satellite platform control centers that migrate to destination locations to repair and upgrade cells and organs. Redundant processors provide real-time data-processing and distribute the data throughout the body with the help of some seven trillion glycans and glycoproteins per drop of blood.

We have proved that increasing the amount of certain intellectual carbohydrates in the body can improve performance of cell ladder logic capabilities and greater athletic abilities. More is better. More glycans, glycoproteins, and glycolipids in the human body will optimize its function for more reach, speed, precision and sometimes even to halt the death process.

In our Glycoscience Medical Conferences case studies are a part of our educational format and are well documented. The Case Studies outlined here do not mention the individuals by name nor the medical institutes.

Halt the Death Process Case Studies

There are several case studies where the patient survived with "Halt the Death Process" and fully recovered from the death sentence that the doctors said was within hours or days at the most.

I will simply call these two Case Studies #1 and #2 and refrain from using the full names of patients, doctors, and major medical facilities.

Cast Study #1
Perhaps the first Case ever in America of a newborn baby who received Smart Sugars via a feeding tube.

Hollis was born October 16, 1997 and was diagnosed with Neonatal

Disseminated Herpes one week after birth. A team of doctors gave "no hope" for Hollis. This terminal illness had taken the life of every baby previously born with his condition in this well known prestigious medical facility. Because the doctors "knew" there was no hope, they told the mother and father to "*Let him die.*" It was explained to the parents that if Hollis lived he would be a vegetable with no brain. And his vital organs were not working. **Hollis was given three days to live.**

Testing and more testing continued. Among other complications, it was concluded that Hollis had a terminal liver condition.

I remember getting a call from the father pleading for help. "*Can you call our doctor?*" For legal reasons I told the father that I could not, but his doctor was welcome to call us. The doctor called and spoke to a physician who was also one of our co-pioneers of Glycoscience.

"*We cannot give anything that is not on our FDA-Approved list of prescribed drugs,*" was the standard echo. However, Smart Sugars were allowed through Hollis' feeding tube because of the determination of the father. He had to sign a waiver indemnifying the hospital of all responsibility. Hollis' condition had not improved or changed in a positive way. The doctors acknowledged that all known medical procedures had been exhausted.

Within five days of Hollis receiving the Smart Sugars, the jaundice yellow color of his skin had totally disappeared.

The doctor ordered a sonogram of his liver. The father watched the doctor looking intently at the monitor and asked, "*What do you see?*" There was a long silence. After several minutes, the father added, "*How does it look?*"

The older grey-haired doctor finally replied, "*I don't know. I've never seen anything like this before.*" The father inched closer to the monitor. There, he witnessed with his own eyes what transfixed the doctor. There were tiny flashes of sparkles of lights in the liver. It was evident that his liver was beginning to function because he was now no longer jaundice.

The bewildered doctor added, "*We don't do sonograms on corpses, and I have never seen a liver revive from such a deadened state.*"

Over the next six weeks the swelling went down and the obvious healing process was thrilling. The doctors who were cautious and negative began to be visibly encouraged, quite positive, and even upbeat.

The death process was halted long enough by the Smart Sugars by supplying needed energy to his cells. His little, horribly bloated yellow body was responding to the energy and his immune system came online.

The day final came when Hollis and his parents could take him home. For another six months, he would be tube fed, first through the nose and mouth, then through a button placed on his stomach. Later they returned to the medical center to have his feeding tube removed.

Yearly checkups proved a delight for the staff at the hospital as they testified to his progress. Tests showed no disorder at all. At eighteen months, they said his mental development was that of a two year old. He became ahead of his classmates. He began to play musical instruments. Hollis became quite athletic. In October of this year (2017) he is a healthy active 20 years old.

Personal Note: My wife, Karen, and I are close friends of Hollis' family. You can imagine the joy of hugging Hollis' neck two decades later. WOW!!! Thank God!

Disclaimer: During the traumatic early days of the life of Hollis, family and friends prayed and sang to him before he was born and at his bedside in the ICU. That may account for his love of music. And it may account for his "impossible" recovery.

Side Comment: It was reported that every baby born in that hospital pre and post Hollis with the same disease, has died. Only Hollis lived. This punctuates the ever so slow change the medical establishment is willing to make, even though the results are clearly self-evident. The FDA still requires that the LD_{50} Level must be met. **The results are millions of unnecessary deaths.**

Case Study #2:

Adult male. I will call him Greg.

Greg (44) was a well known executive of a famous company in a major US city. He was not feeling well. In fact, he knew something was seriously wrong. He developed a sore throat a few weeks earlier. But, now the aches and pains became so serious that he checked himself into the hospital. His temperature was 107 degrees. Within hours of his arrival at the hospital, everything with the scope of traditional medical help had been done.

The diagnosis was streptococceeal toxic-shock syndrome. The doctors could not stabilize Greg. Instead, his vital organs were failing.

By the following morning, he was deteriorating literally by the minute. The family was called and instructed that there was no hope and that they should expect the worst. The doctor in charge had basic education in Glycoscience. He told the family that there may be a way to halt the death process long enough to allow the body to begin healing but it was a long-shot without any guarantee. The family said, "*Do it!*"

The doctor later told us that Greg's condition was so extreme that every cell of his body was affected. Greg received twenty-five grams of the Smart Sugars through his feeding tube every four hours.

Within a few hours his doctor recorded that Greg had turned the corner. He left the hospital whole except for a kidney that was later donated by his brother. Greg enjoyed a productive life for five years when he died from a heart attack.

Source and References:

http://Glycosciencewhitepaper.com

Expand Your Mind - Improve Your Brain http://endowmentmed.org/content/view/826/106/

Change Your Sugar, Change Your Life http://DiabeticHope.com

Glycoscience Lesson #50 http://GlycoscienceNEWS.com/pdf/Lesson50.pdf

http://EzineArticles.com/?expert=JC_Spencer

© The Endowment for Medical Research http://endowmentmed.org

Chapter Six

A Brief Look at Quantum Glycoscience

Einstein called quantum physics,
"spooky action at a distance."

**Today's scientists believe
quantum physics challenges
Einstein's Theory of Relativity.**

Quantum biology is an emerging science discipline. Quantum Glycobiology or Quantum Glycoscience (QG) will help us solve the mysteries of why some sugars are so unbelievably beneficial for improving health and may enable us to correct otherwise impossible devastating illnesses.

Quantum science was, even for Albert Einstein, a hard pill to swallow because of its mind bending, paradoxical explanation of phenomena. Today, a little bit of sugar will, that's right, help make the medicine go down.

Scientists are grasping at quantum's bizarre properties to solve mysteries of the evident influence of unseen forces. We will learn how to harness quantum influences; but, first we need to understand how the same wave-particle properties can produce drastically different outcomes.

There is yet much to learn concerning the three known glycoforms. The three known glycoforms on or in our cells are glycans, glycoproteins, and glycolipids.

Before we can best understand QG, we need to discover the unknown influences and the known influences that we do not see but can measure. But first, it may benefit our readers to have a very short lesson in proteins.

Proteomics

Proteomics cover a range of disciplines concerning the structure and function of proteins in the biological systems. In the 1980s, proteins were the focus of much research. It was a shock to some of my glycoscience pioneers when Dr Bill McAnalley discovered that the functional component in aloe vera was a carbohydrate instead of a protein. I will explain HOW he made that discovery in a moment.

Günter Blobel, recipient of the Nobel Prize in Proteomics in 1999 was for discovery of signals that govern transport and localization in the cell. Dr. Blobel mentioned glycoproteins in his research conducted in 1982 but his focus was on the proteins. Scientists thought proteins were the main functional component. Proteomics received the credit for the signals instead of glycomics because little was known about glycobiology at the time. The term, "glycobiology" was not coined until 1988 at Oxford University.

It will be beneficial if we better understand what is the criteria for properly folding proteins. We know that the structural folding of proteins is determined by or actually conformed according to the needed function. The "random" coiling of proteins may not be random at all. There is cause and effect for every fold or twist and turn of the proteins that are continually manufactured at lightening speed throughout the human body.

The challenge to understand protein folding is multiplied by incorporating the Smart Sugars into the entanglement. The angle of the bonds at each juncture is significant. Sugars that are responsible for proper folding of the proteins include Trehalose in conjunction with other sugars to help carry out the assignment for properly folding of the proteins.

Glycomics

Glycomics cover a range of disciplines concerning the structure and function of carbohydrates in the biological systems.

Dr Bill McAnalley, toxicologist and pharmacologist, was the first scientist to discover a medicinal benefit from a sugar. He was expecting to discover a certain protein as the healing agent. The story goes that as he was working in his lab in Arlington, Texas when there was a power failure. He had a small power backup system which supplied electricity for a light and small microwave oven. He told me that in frustration, he tossed some aloe vera into the microwave to nuke it. He soon learned that the functional component was NOT destroyed by the microwave. Had it been a protein, it would have indeed been nuked. Dr. McAnalley knew then that it was a carbohydrate and learned soon thereafter that the functional sugar was mannose.

The trillion dollar question is how to properly fold the proteins. Perhaps all this entanglement with unknown forces makes anything possible with quantum mechanics. In Quantum Glycoscience, it will be necessary to understand how the folding of different proteins and sugars are orchestrated by variant thermal conditions, light of various spectrums, rate of radioactive decay, direction of rotation, speed of spin, angle of molecular bonds, strength of molecular bond, gravity, electrical discharge transfer of energy, ions, magnetism, photons, radiation, and thought.

I could hear you whisper, *"How can thought be involved in quantum glyco-biology?"* Think! In clinical studies, the placebo effect works on about a third of the patients who are taking a sugar pill, a "bad sugar" pill yet. Animals don't exhibit the placebo effect.

It was the variant factors of entanglement that baffled Einstein and caused him to call quantum physics, *"spooky action at a distance."* The real relativity factor of future science is to better understand the entanglement. The reason the entanglement factor is so important is the fact that it often works at the tipping point of change. The tipping point factor can be explained with a perfectly balanced virtual scale holding in each bucket half the water of all the oceans. The tipping point for the scale to tilt either direction is determined by adding one drop of water to your choice of either side. This is how relative a drop of H_2O is when it puts its weight behind a purpose.

In quantum physics, the possibilities are endless, not just one tilting to the left or right like the drop of water on the scale. The endless possibilities of mysterious influences can alter the state and performance of a molecule or a system. The effect, the behavior, the consequences, are as pervasive as they are profound.

Quantum influences are relative to all systems regardless of size. Quantum physicists have been concerned primarily with microscopic anomalies. There may be no boundaries of quantum prediction because of the incoherence of unknown factors. It is this entanglement that binds all the particles together to produce unknown quantities for conclusions of which some may manifest as very strange and surprising. Here collective properties seemingly become impossible to untangle. However, we need to reverse engineer the folding. To understand the unfolding in slow motion may provide answers that will effect how we deal with longevity and health for mankind.

Like the tilted scale, when the propensity is altered, that newly directed influence may gather momentum and influence compounding change. I postulate that the peer pressure of particle momentum influences atoms, ions, photons, magnetism, and thought. In fact, a thought triggers a constellation of synapses in your brain to take flight like a flock of birds. Scientists have learned that elementary particles also react like waves of activity and develop a propensity to operate in unison. This is the law of influence. The influence which may be to attract or repel.

It is the very entanglement that produces the outcome. Mangled entanglement produces chaos. It is the proper folding of proteins that gives order to the human body and the misfolding of these same proteins that causes or accentuates all neurodegenerative diseases.

Quantum glycobiology resides in the entanglement of proteins and sugars forming glycan, glycolipids and glycoproteins that are the Operating System (OS) of the human body.

Like Sands of the Sea or Stars of the Constellations

Consider some 800,000 glycans and glycoproteins on just one cell. Then consider some 70 trillion cells in the human body. Add to that, the consideration of the many bonds and branches of various long chain polysaccharides and various proteins in each glycoform. Now, consider the angle of each bond and the strength of each bond. Taking all of this into consideration, Glycoscience is more complex than the genome project.

Why Quantum Glycoscience IS the Future of Medicine

The needed research in QG will provide many medical students with his or her doctoral thesis. It is in the many imperfections of glycosylation that we will find the cause for or the accentuation of ALL DISEASES.

Vlatko Vedral of Oxford admits, "*Implications of macroscopic objects such as us being in quantum limbo is mind blowing enough that we physicists are still in an entangled state of confusion and wonderment .*"

It appears no one understands quantum physics; yet, that has not kept brilliant minds from enjoying the possibilities nor kept them from babbling utter nonsense about things that are not even relative. Quantum physics extend new opposing challenges to the theory of relativity. And, QG opens the door for understanding the benefits of Smart Sugars like never before. Meanwhile, the efficacy of these Smart Sugars is self-evident. You are not required to understand the science to enjoy its benefits.

Funding for Quantum Glycoscience Research

Our vision at the GLYCOSCIENCE INSTITUTE and the TEXAS ENDOWMENT FOR MEDICAL RESEARCH is to help supply select medical students with scholarship opportunities in the discipline of Quantum Glycoscience. This program may hold significant breakthroughs to minimize, reverse, or complete eliminate various diseases.

Funding for QG Research has the most results oriented potential in medical research. We will expand our collaboration with universities and medical schools with opportunities to establish Quantum Glycoscience Departments. We will provide the blueprints for dozens of research programs from which the medical students may choose. The select students will be provided a choice of QG Research Projects from which they can earn their degrees.

Yes, without question, Quantum Glycoscience is the future of medicine and healthcare. The medical possibilities of QG is without limit and will indeed forever change the way we live.

Many American Veterans are cast
along the side of the road like rag dolls
by the bureaucratic process.

Chaos in medical and healthcare
is because of ignorance, greed,
mismanagement, and neglect.

Similarities abound for treating
trauma for military warriors
and civil warrior athletes.

It is A Time for Truth.
It is A Time for Action.
It is A Time for RESULTS.

Chapter Seven

Make the VA Great Again and Enable Athletes to Perform and Recover Faster

Military warriors and civil warriors have much in common. The warriors in the military seek to be the best and often suffer mental and physical damage. Athletic warriors seek to be the best they can be and often suffer mental and physical damage. Concussions, broken bones, and torn ligaments often result in long term bodily and emotional damage.

Similarities in treating trauma for military warriors and civil warrior athletes are virtually parallel.

In 2003, Four-Star Marine General Raymond Davis and I planned to mobilize veterans to declare war on a domestic enemy, but...

General Raymond Davis was America's most decorated hero. His battles were in World War II, the Korean War, and the Vietnam Conflict. Presidents under whom he served included Harry S Truman, Dwight D Eisenhower, John F Kennedy, Lyndon B Johnson, Richard M Nixon, Gerald Ford, George H W Bush, and Ronald Reagan.

In this chapter I will discuss how he and I met and what was to be his next battle. And, I will discuss a new battle against a serious domestic enemy to be fought in his name.

Every American Veteran is invited to join and fight this enemy that has millions of Americans in its grasp. The fight is against Post-traumatic stress disorder (PTSD) and psychotropic drugs that often compound the problems.

It is A Time for Truth. It is A Time for Action. It is A Time for Self-Evident Results.

It is time that each of us, including every able veteran, take charge of their own health and demand results instead of acquiescing for someone else to fix the problem.

Ignorance is overcome with knowledge and the wisdom to know what to do with the knowledge.

Greed is overcome with a caring heart for others. Mismanagement is overcome with skills that are trained to produce results.

Neglect is overcome by leadership with purpose that exchanges greed for compassion and mismanagement with proper training;

One of the biggest concerns for the veterans is neurological damage that strains the mental and motor skills.

Let us Address PTSD NOW! Current Efforts are Failing

Post-traumatic stress disorder (PTSD) is a serious challenge with the neurological system. PTSD is triggered by memories of a stressful event that bring a level of anxiety that can cause intense fear and feelings of helplessness. PTSD can be triggered simply by observing a traumatic event. PTSD may persist long after the event. It is estimated that more than five million adults in the United States are affected by PTSD each year.

"Experts" are not sure what causes some people to develop PTSD more seriously than others. Your brain processes thoughts and feelings differently from anyone else. Scientists studying the brain observe that all brains are differences in the brain structure and chemistry. Certain areas of the brain involved with feeling and fear are more hyperactive in some people. This may contribute to PTSD.

Treatments for PTSD often includes:

Conventional psychotherapy by a psychotherapist reported to be one of the main treatments for PTSD. The purpose is to manage thoughts and feelings of the traumatic event with cognitive behavior therapy (CBT). The idea is to develop tolerance for the fears. The goal of CBT is equipt the PTSD patient to control fear and anxiety.

Stress management therapy that teaches relaxation techniques in an attempt to break the cycle of negative thoughts.

Medication and prayer

Without question, these treatments when properly administered can be very beneficial; however that may not resolve the issues of PTSD and drastic therapies are called for.

Drastic measures of drug therapies is like throwing mud on a wall to see if it sticks.

The urgent attempt to correct PTSD often causes more problems than solutions.

Drug treatments for PTSD include:

Antidepressants for selective serotonin reuptake inhibitors (SSRIs), including sertraline (Zoloft), fluoxetine (Prozac), fluvoxamine (Luvox), or paroxetine (Paxil).

Benzodiazepines for sedating, including lorazepam (Ativan) and alprazolam (Xanax).

Dopamine-blocking agents (neuroleptics)

Other means of Therapies for PTSD include:

Several mind-body techniques including Eye Movement Desensitization and Reprocessing (EMDR), in which the patient moves his or her eyes rapidly from side to side while recalling the traumatic event. This seems to help reduce distress for some with PTSD. Doctors do not understand how it works or how long PTSD symptoms are reduced using EMDR.

Biofeedback involves using a drug to see bodily functions that are normally unconscious and occur involuntarily. As the body reacts to stress, the patient learns to perform certain techniques to eventually control the reactions without using the biofeedback machine. Some studies indicate that biofeedback may be an effective treatment.

Hypnosis has been used to treat war-related post-traumatic conditions by inducing a deep state of relaxation so the patient feels safer. Hypnosis is normally used with or by a psychotherapist.

Emotional Freedom Technique (EFT) is a process that combines tapping on acupuncture points while calling to mind traumatic events. Anecdotal evidence with PTSD patients has been encouraging.

Acupuncture has helped with symptoms of PTSD including insomnia, anxiety, and depression.

Nutrition is a do and don't protocol that includes eliminating certain foods to which the patient may be allergic. Certain foods and drinks that fall into this category are stimulants such as coffee, alcohol, tobacco, and too much sugar especially in soft drinks. An improved diet is always welcomed by the body and brain.

Scientists are aiming at the urgent while neglecting the important. Symptoms are treated in impossible efforts to stop the bleeding. The immediate need is understanding what makes our neurological system work, how the signals communicate, and what we can do to improve brain function.

A part of the secret to the neurological system is proper glycosylation of the cells. This can be accomplished through Glycoscience and the application of Smart Sugars technology which is proved to be save and effective.

Our veterans are treated with toxic drugs when new technology is available but not used. Four-Star Marine General Raymond Davis and I had a battle plan that was ended when he died of a heart attack on September 3, 2003 at the age of 88. He was considered our most decorated General.

Today, in memory of General Raymond Davis, we have a new VA Cause. Every American Veteran is invited to join and we need commanding leaders to fight a domestic enemy. PTSD is to adults what ADHD is to some young people.

What an honor it was for me to have him accept the vision and desire to go into one more battle. What a man! What a General! A list of his medals and decorations include: the Medal of Honor; the Navy Cross; the Distinguished Service Medal with Gold Star in lieu of a second award; the Silver Star Medal with Gold Star in lieu of a second award; the Legion of Merit with Combat "V" and Gold Star in lieu of a second award; the Bronze Star Medal with Combat "V"; the Purple Heart; the Presidential Unit Citation with four bronze stars indicative of second through fifth awards; the Navy Unit Commendation; the American Defense Service Medal with Fleet clasp; the American Campaign Medal; the Asiatic-Pacific Campaign Medal with one silver star in lieu of five bronze stars; the World War II Victory Medal; the National Defense Service Medal with one bronze star; the Korean Service Medal with four bronze stars; the Vietnam Service Medal with three bronze stars; the National Order of Vietnam, 4th Class; the National Order of Vietnam, 4th Class; the Vietnamese Cross of Gallantry with three Palms; two Korean Presidential Unit Citations; the United Nations Service Medal; and the Republic of Vietnam Campaign Medal.

I'm asking every veteran and friends and families of a veteran join forces to fight the Domestic Enemy of Psychotropic Drugs in Honor of General Raymond Davis.

Psychotropic Drugs to Treat Attention-Deficit/ Hyperactivity Disorder (ADHD) may be Domestic Enemies as are some Drugs used to Treat PTSD.

An American Veteran's national campaign against psychotropic drugs was forming in 2003. I was asked to design the campaign with Four-Star Marine General Raymond Davis. The declared domestic enemy was damaging the minds, emotions, and behavior of our children.

My good friend Jim Cabaniss, founder of American Veterans In Domestic Defense (AVIDD), introduced me to General Davis. We were excited about his eagerness to champion the cause. He would help save many children by leading the fight and recruiting an all volunteer army of veterans.

Our PR campaign would use various action phrases such as: **Join General Raymond Davis in his final battle to save America's Children**. "Ray" Davis was our most decorated hero. His other battles were in World War II, the Korean War, and the Vietnam Conflict. His commanding officers were Truman, Eisenhower, Kennedy, Johnson, Nixon, Ford, Bush, and Reagan.

Each person in the military had already pledged to defend America against every enemy, foreign and domestic. The campaign for General Davis to lead American Veterans into battle against this domestic enemy would be victorious; however, Ray suffered a heart attack and died on August 6, 2003 at the age of 88.

Today the Investigative Journalist Alan Schwarz is fighting the battle against psychotropic drugs through his book, ADHD Nation. Schwarz was the author of the book and documentary, Head Game, which brought to light concussions in sports that result in brain injuries, drug abuse and suicidal thoughts. Concussion, the major 2015 motion picture, exposed the NFL coverup that resulted in deaths of some players. Scores of deceased NFL players were found to have brain disease.

In the book ADHD Nation, Alan Schwarz calls ADHD misdiagnosis **"a national disaster of dangerous proportions."** Some legal drugs given to our children are as dangerous as cocaine and have lifelong consequences. He believes that perhaps two-thirds of the children diagnosed with ADHD are not ADHD. His book is a damning indictment of the pharmaceutical industry and clearly outlines what is damaging our youth in the name of mental health. Schwarz sees big pharma using academic pressures on our young people and their families.

Of course, big pharma is defending the indefensible and denies the undeniable that children are trading these legal drugs in schools, that there are vast numbers of misdiagnosis cases, and that the CDC could not be right in their evaluations. The CDC reported in 2013 that approximately 6% of U.S. adolescents aged 12 – 19 use psychotropic drugs and 3.2% use antidepressants.

The simple fact is that harmful sugars in food and drinks produce or compound ADHD like symptoms. Another simple fact is that Smart Sugars have a very positive affect while improving brain function. We were excited to participate in a sugar research in Israel with the conclusion that the One Smart Sugar - Trehalose was actually an anti-depressant.

Source and References:

https://www.scientificamerican.com/article/big-pharma-s-manufactured-epidemic-the-misdiagnosis-of-adhd/

Change Your Sugar, Change Your Life http://DiabeticHope.com

http://OneSmartSsugar.com

Expand Your Mind - Improve Your Brain http://endowmentmed.org/content/view/826/106/

Glycoscience Lesson #48 http://GlycoscienceNEWS.com/pdf/Lesson48.pdf

http://EzineArticles.com/?expert=JC_Spencer

© **The Endowment for Medical Research** http://endowmentmed.org

Chapter Eight

Leading Doctors Verify That Integrating Glycoscience Has Self-Evident Benefits

**TV commercials are educating
the general public about drugs
that your doctor may
know nothing about.**

**My favorite commercial
ends something like,
*"After taking the drug,
if you go blind and deaf,
consult your doctor."***

Ben Carson, MD is known around the world for breakthroughs in neurosurgery that have brought hope where there was no hope. Barbara Walter on ABC News said, "*He works miracles on children others have written off as hopeless.*"

Dr Carson was director of the division of neurosurgery, oncology, plastic surgery, and pediatric neurosurgery, and a professor of neurosurgery, oncology, plastic surgery, and pediatrics at the Johns Hopkins Medical Institutes. He holds more than forty honorary doctorate degrees and numerous other awards.

His knowledge of the benefits of Smart Sugars was learned from a young patient who was recovering better than others patients following neural surgery. This encounter would play a significant role in his own health.

Not only did Dr Carson develop prostate cancer, but the biopsy indicated a very malignant and aggressive form. After talking with one of my close pioneering medical doctor friends about Smart Sugars, he reviewed some of the scientific studies behind the sugars. Of course, he recognized that regular sugar feeds cancer, however these specific sugars were beneficial against cancer. He then began ingesting the specific sugars.

Dr Carson gave serious consideration to forgo the medical options and to use only [Smart Sugars] instead. Smart Sugars seemed like a promising natural remedy. But he decided to consider the risk of what others might do if they followed his example should the alternative route fail for them. He literally put others before himself in his decision and opted for traditional surgery integrated with Smart Sugars.

Knowledge of applied Glycoscience became such a strong influence on Dr Carson's life that he wrote about his battle with aggressive prostate cancer in his book <u>Take the Risk</u> Chapter 13 "*My Personal Risks in the Face of Death.*"

Dr Carson was the keynote speaker for our 2006 Glycoscience Medical Conference in Houston and he later taught a Glycoscience TV program for the Public Broadcasting System (PBS).

The PBS fund raising program with Dr Ben Carson on Glycoscience was first tested in the Phoenix market. The report I received was that this proved more successful in raising funds than any program they had ever conducted. It was used in a few other television markets for PBS. When he entered the Presidential race, the training was no longer aired. Now that he is in the Trump administration, it is doubtful PBS will continue to air his Glycoscience training any time soon.

Many physicians are learning more about immunology through Glycoscience and integrating this knowledge into their practices. Some of my friends were threatened with losing their licenses. Some quietly served a short time in federal prison for curing cancer. It was a powerful lesson that we cannot treat or cure anyone without an approved drug procedure. A good medical doctor friend nearly lost his license because of his success in overcoming AIDS in patients with Smart Sugars.

Rayburne Goen, MD was a family physician in Tulsa for about sixty years. His wife had passed and he was at the end of his life with twenty-one health challenges. After he learned about Glycoscience, he applied the Smart Sugars to his daily regimen. Within four months, twenty of the twenty-one ailments were gone and he was "his old self" again.

Dr Goen had a patient from the time she was born fifty years earlier with a neurological challenge. She was unable to feed herself, comb her hair, and brush her teeth. For fifty years, she was in bed or in a chair or wheelchair. Dr Goen knew there was no toxicity in the Smart Sugars and that they were safe and would have no negative side effects. He started her on a Smart Sugar regimen.

At one of our Glycoscience Medical Conferences shortly before he died at the age of 94, Dr Goen, himself, was a case study and also presented his observation of his patient of fifty years.

My wife and I have a painting in our livingroom that we bought from Dr Goen because... After a few months ingesting Smart Sugars, Dr Goen's patient of fifty years, not only started brushing her teeth, combing her hair, and feeding herself – she painted a three-dimensional shadow box picture. It is one of our most treasured possessions we have in our home.

Chapter Nine

Change is Coming!
Change is Inevitable!
And, it can be very very good.

Congress can save US Trillions of Dollars, make great medical advancements, and greatly benefit the people with better health and healthcare:

Pass a new Law to restructure the FDA. Also, fund another Law already on the Books that was intentionally never funded. And, make DSHEA (Dietary Supplement Health and Education Act of 1994) and the Office of Dietary Supplements independent from the FDA.

DSHEA
Dietary Supplement Health and Education Act

This story is one of politicians big deceptions.

The Law and the Plan for Better Health Worldwide. – Put on the books and intentionally never funded. The public thought Congress passed this into Law unanimously. That was the PR behind the new Law.

Since DSHEA was passed into Law in 1994

The DSHEA law was enacted because consumers were outraged when the US Congress moved to remove consumer access to nutritional supplements. Public furor mobilized Congress to pass DSHEA with what appeared to be unanimous Congressional consent.

Contrary to popular belief, in 1994, DSHEA did not pass by a unanimous vote on the floor of the House and the Senate.

According to Loren Israelsen and Thomas D. Aarts in an article published in *Nutrition Business Journal* entitled "DSHEA Ten Years Later: Now What?", no floor vote on DSHEA was ever held in the House. In fact, they say, that the House version of DSHEA never even made it out of committee. DSHEA became law because of a "perfect storm" confluence of political forces.

Israelsen and Aarts said that the Gingrich New Deal Republicans were about to sweep out the old line House Democrats who were holding up DSHEA, which caused the Democrats to unload the DSHEA issue at the very last minute to save their jobs. In the Senate, Senator Orrin Hatch (R-UT) was able to hold off a last minute attempt to derail DSHEA as it was coming up for unanimous consent vote in the closing minutes of the 1994 Senate session.

Literally, DSHEA was a political "Hail Mary" of unprecedented proportions. Apparently, frantic last-minute deal making resulted in the addition of the structure/ function claim disclaimer, among some other last minute changes.

Since passage in 1994, the industry has pacified itself into believing that DSHEA was an overwhelming political victory (indeed, it was) because it was unanimously voted for by the Congress (which it was not). DSHEA was created by last minute deals. Last minute deal making is the way of the political process.

By making DSHEA the global standard, the economics of countries can be impacted. In the US alone, delaying the onset of Alzheimer's Disease one year can save the nation four hundred fifty billion dollars ($450,000,000,000)* in assisted care costs for just Alzheimer's disease patients.

Many deadly diseases could be eliminated from the planet by making DSHEA the standard for nutrients. DSHEA is a unique pro-health US law that treats nutrients as foods, which indeed they are. Nutrients are safe and effective and have important clinical impact in preventing, mitigating, treating, and curing diseases from under-nutrition.

DSHEA is the counter to the pro-illness impact of standards and guidelines of Codex. Perhaps the greatest single impediment to advancing health to the world is the Codex Alimentarius Commission (CAC, or Codex). The restrictive Codex Vitamin and Mineral Guideline (VMG, ratified July 4, 2005, Rome) treats vitamins and minerals as toxins whose upper limits must be determined by "risk assessment" (RA), a technique used in toxicology to determine the highest dose of a poison that can be given to a human being without any discernible impact. The VMG limits upper doses of nutrients to levels that do not exceed those found in unprocessed food. Since ubiquitous and specific toxins increase the need for nutrients, this short-sighted and dangerous Codex text both mandates and institutionalizes deadly levels of under-nutrition.

Codex employs a double standard that favors corporate interests by permitting extraordinarily high health-adverse levels of dangerous toxins like pesticides, veterinary drugs, synthetic growth hormones, heavy metals, preservatives, and food additives.

Many of Codex's more than 5,000 standards and guidelines degrade the integrity of the food supply and health. Two groups, The Natural Solutions Foundation and Citizen's Codex Working Group, have crafted a comprehensive strategy that allows nations to protect their people from toxins and under-nutrition while avoiding World Trade Organization (WTO) trade sanctions.

What they call, the "Codex 2-Step," can be applied by pro-health countries to any of the damaging or dangerous standards and guidelines promulgated by Codex.

Once a country has adopted a revised and more scientifically valid standard or guideline than that required within a Codex text:

(Step 1) It must then enact national legislation to make revised standard or guideline becomes national law

(Step 2). Having carried out the required two-step process, the country is then free to engage in the manufacture and trade (including export) of items that would otherwise be prohibited by the Codex standards and guidelines. For example, the sale of high-potency nutritional supplements permitted under a DSHEA-type law currently violates the restrictive and deadly Codex VMG. The Natural Solutions Foundation helps countries establish access to unlimited amounts of dietary supplements at their discretion by establishing the principles of DSHEA globally.

* *The figure $450,000,000,000 is considerably less than the author's estimation of $1,000,000,000,000 as outlined in Chapter Two.*

Dietary Supplement Health and Education Act of 1994
Public Law 103-417
103rd Congress

An Act

To amend the Federal Food, Drug, and Cosmetic Act to establish standards with respect to dietary supplements, and for other purposes.

Be it enacted by the Senate and House of Representatives of the United States of America in Congress assembled,

§1. Short Title; Reference; Table Of Contents.

(a) Short Title.
>This Act may be cited as the "Dietary Supplement Health and Education Act of 1994".

(b) Reference.
>Whenever in this Act an amendment or repeal is expressed in terms of an amendment to, or repeal of, a section or other provision, the reference shall be considered to be made to a section or other provision of the Federal Food, Drug, and Cosmetic Act.

(c) Table of Contents.
>The table of contents of this Act is as follows:

§2. Findings.

Congress finds that -
(1)   **improving the health status of United States citizens ranks at the top of the national priorities of the Federal Government;**
(2)   **the importance of nutrition and the benefits of dietary supplements to health promotion and disease prevention have been documented increasingly in scientific studies;**
(3)   **(A)**   **there is a link between the ingestion of certain nutrients or dietary supplements and the prevention of chronic diseases such as cancer, heart disease, and osteoporosis; and**
         (B)   **clinical research has shown that several chronic diseases can be prevented simply with a healthful diet, such as a diet that is low in fat, saturated fat, cholesterol, and sodium, with a high proportion of plant-based foods;**
(4)   **healthful diets may mitigate the need for expensive medical procedures, such as coronary bypass surgery or angioplasty;**

(5)   **preventive health measures, including education, good nutrition, and appropriate use of safe nutritional supplements will limit the incidence of chronic diseases, and reduce long-term health care expenditures;**
(6)   **(A)**   **promotion of good health and healthy lifestyles improves and extends lives while reducing health care expenditures; and**
         (B)   **reduction in health care expenditures is of paramount importance to the future of the country and the economic well-being of the country;**
(7)   **there is a growing need for emphasis on the dissemination of information linking nutrition and long-term good health;**
(8)   **consumers should be empowered to make choices about preventive health care programs based on data from**

scientific studies of health benefits related to particular dietary supplements;

(9)   national surveys have revealed that almost 50 percent of the 260,000,000 Americans regularly consume dietary supplements of vitamins, minerals, or herbs as a means of improving their nutrition;

(10)   studies indicate that consumers are placing increased reliance on the use of nontraditional health care providers to avoid the excessive costs of traditional medical services and to obtain more holistic consideration of their needs;

(11)   the United States will spend over $1,000,000,000,000 on health care in 1994, which is about 12 percent of the Gross National Product of the United States, and this amount and percentage will continue to increase unless significant efforts are undertaken to reverse the increase;

(12)   (A)   the nutritional supplement industry is an integral part of the economy of the United States;

        (B)   the industry consistently projects a positive trade balance; and

        (C)   the estimated 600 dietary supplement manufacturers in the United States produce approximately 4,000 products, with total annual sales of such products alone reaching at least $4,000,000,000;

(13)   although the Federal Government should take swift action against products that are unsafe or adulterated, the Federal Government should not take any actions to impose unreasonable regulatory barriers limiting or slowing the flow of safe products and accurate information to consumers;

(14)   dietary supplements are safe within a broad range of intake, and safety problems with the supplements are relatively rare; and

(15)   (A)   legislative action that protects the right of access of consumers to safe dietary supplements is necessary in order to promote wellness; and

        (B)   a rational Federal framework must be established to supersede the current ad hoc, patchwork regulatory policy on dietary supplements.

§3. Definitions.

    (a) Definition of Certain Foods as Dietary Supplements. Section 201 (21 U.S.C. 321) is amended by adding at the end the following:

        "(ff) The term "dietary supplement" -

            "(1)   means a product (other than tobacco) intended to supplement the diet that bears or contains one or more of the following dietary ingredients:

                "(A)   a vitamin;

                "(B)   a mineral;

                "(C)   an herb or other botanical;

                "(D)   an amino acid;

                "(E)   a dietary substance for use by man to supplement the diet by increasing the total dietary intake; or

                "(F)   a concentrate, metabolite, constituent, extract, or combination of any ingredient described in clause (A), (B), (C), (D), or (E);

            "(2)   means a product that -

                "(A)   (I)   is intended for ingestion in a form described in section 411(c)(1)(B)(i); or "(ii) complies with section 411(c)(1)(B)(ii);

                "(B)   is not represented for use as a conventional food or as a sole item of a meal or the diet; and

                "(C)   is labeled as a dietary supplement; and

            "(3) does -

                "(A)   include an article that is approved as a new drug under section 505, certified as an antibiotic under section 507, or licensed as a biologic under section 351 of the Public Health Service Act (42 U.S.C. 262) and was, prior to such approval, certification, or license, marketed as a dietary supplement or as a food unless the Secretary has issued a regulation, after notice and comment, finding that the article, when used as or in a dietary supplement under the conditions of use and dosages set forth in the labeling for such dietary supplement, is unlawful under section 402(f); and

"(B) not include -

"(I)   an article that is approved as a new drug under section 505, certified as an antibiotic under section 507, or licensed as a biologic under section 351 of the Public Health Service Act (42 U.S.C. 262), or

"(ii)   an article authorized for investigation as a new drug, antibiotic, or biological for which substantial clinical investigations have been instituted and for which the existence of such investigations has been made public, which was not before such approval, certification, licensing, or authorization marketed as a dietary supplement or as a food unless the Secretary, in the Secretary's discretion, has issued a regulation, after notice and comment, finding

that the article would be
lawful under this Act.

Except for purposes of section 201(g), a
dietary supplement shall be deemed to
be a food within the meaning of this
Act.

(b)   **Exclusion from Definition of Food Additive.**
Section 201(s) (21 U.S.C. 321(s)) is amended -
(1)   by striking "or" at the end of
subparagraph (4);
(2)   by striking the period at the end of
subparagraph (5) and inserting "; or";
and
(3)   by adding at the end the following new
subparagraph (6) "an ingredient
described in paragraph (ff) in, or
intended for use in, a dietary
supplement.".

(c)   **Form of Ingestion.** Section 411(c)(1)(B) (21
U.S.C. 350(c)(1)(B)) is amended -
(1)   in clause (i), by inserting "powder,
softgel, gelcap," after "capsule,"; and
(2)   in clause (ii), by striking "does not
simulate and".

§4. Safety of Dietary Supplements and Burden of Proof on FDA.
Section 402 (21 U.S.C. 342) is amended by adding at the end the
following:

"(f)(1) If it is a dietary supplement or contains a dietary ingredient
that -
"(A) presents a significant or unreasonable risk of illness or
injury under -
"(i) conditions of use recommended or suggested in
labeling, or
"(ii) if no conditions of use are suggested or

recommended in the labeling, under ordinary conditions of use;

"(B) is a new dietary ingredient for which there is inadequate information to provide reasonable assurance that such ingredient does not present a significant or unreasonable risk of illness or injury;

"(C) the Secretary declares to pose an imminent hazard to public health or safety, except that the authority to make such declaration shall not be delegated and the Secretary shall promptly after such a declaration initiate a proceeding in accordance with sections 554 and 556 of title 5, United States Code, to affirm or withdraw the declaration; or

"(D) is or contains a dietary ingredient that renders it adulterated under paragraph (a)(1) under the conditions of use recommended or suggested in the labeling of such dietary supplement.

In any proceeding under this subparagraph, **the United States shall bear the burden of proof on each element to show that a dietary supplement is adulterated.** The court shall decide any issue under this paragraph on a de novo basis.

(2) Before the Secretary may report to a United States attorney a violation of paragraph (1)(A) for a civil proceeding, the person against whom such proceeding would be initiated shall be given appropriate notice and the opportunity to present views, orally and in writing, at least 10 days before such notice, with regard to such proceeding.

§5. Dietary Supplement Claims.
Chapter IV (21 U.S.C. 341 et seq.) is amended by inserting after section 403A the following new section:

DIETARY SUPPLEMENT LABELING EXEMPTIONS

"**Sec. 403B. (a) IN GENERAL.** - A publication, including an article, a chapter in a book, or an official abstract of a peer-reviewed scientific publication that appears in an article and was prepared by the author or the editors of the publication, which is reprinted in its entirety, shall not be defined as labeling when used in connection with the sale of a dietary supplement to consumers when it -

"(1) is not false or misleading;

"(2) does not promote a particular manufacturer or brand of a dietary supplement;

"(3) is displayed or presented, or is displayed or presented with other such items on the same subject matter, so as to present a balanced view of the available scientific information on a dietary supplement;

"(4) if displayed in an establishment, is physically separate from the dietary supplements; and

"(5) does not have appended to it any information by sticker or any other method.

"**(b) APPLICATION.** - Subsection (a) shall not apply to or restrict a retailer or wholesaler of dietary supplements in any way whatsoever in the sale of books or other publications as a part of the business of such retailer or wholesaler.

"**(c) BURDEN OF PROOF.** - In any proceeding brought under subsection (a), the burden of proof shall be on the United States to establish that an article or other such matter is false or misleading.".

§6. Statements of Nutritional Support.

Section 403(r) (21 U.S.C. 343(r)) is amended by adding at the end the following:

"(6) For purposes of paragraph (r)(1)(B), a statement for a dietary supplement may be made if -

> "**(A) the statement claims a benefit related to a classical nutrient deficiency disease and discloses the prevalence of such disease in the United States, describes the role of a nutrient or dietary ingredient intended to affect the structure or function in**

humans, characterizes the documented mechanism by which a nutrient or dietary ingredient acts to maintain such structure or function, or describes general well-being from consumption of a nutrient or dietary ingredient,

"(B) the manufacturer of the dietary supplement has substantiation that such statement is truthful and not misleading, and

"(C) the statement contains, prominently displayed and in boldface type, the following: "This statement has not been evaluated by the Food and Drug Administration. This product is not intended to diagnose, treat, cure, or prevent any disease.".

A statement under this subparagraph may not claim to diagnose, mitigate, treat, cure, or prevent a specific disease or class of diseases. If the manufacturer of a dietary supplement proposes to make a statement described in the first sentence of this subparagraph in the labeling of the dietary supplement, the manufacturer shall notify the Secretary no later than 30 days after the first marketing of the dietary supplement with such statement that such a statement is being made.".

§7. Dietary Supplement Ingredient Labeling and Nutrition Information Labeling.

(a) MISBRANDED SUPPLEMENTS. - Section 403 (21 U.S.C. 343) is amended by adding at the end the following: "(s) If -

"(1) it is a dietary supplement; and

"(2)(A) the label or labeling of the supplement fails to list -

"(i) the name of each ingredient of the supplement that is described in section 201(ff); and

"(ii)(I) the quantity of each such ingredient; or

"(II) with respect to a proprietary blend of such ingredients, the total quantity of all ingredients in the blend;

"(B) the label or labeling of the dietary supplement fails to identify the product by using the term `dietary supplement', which term may be modified with the name of such an ingredient;

"(C) the supplement contains an ingredient described in section 201(ff)(1)(C), and the label or labeling of the supplement fails to identify any part of the plant from which the ingredient is derived;

"(D) the supplement -

"(i) is covered by the specifications of an official compendium;

"(ii) is represented as conforming to the specifications of an official compendium; and

"(iii) fails to so conform; or

"(E) the supplement -

"(i) is not covered by the specifications of an official compendium; and

"(ii)(I) fails to have the identity and strength that the supplement is represented to have; or

"(II) fails to meet the quality (including tablet or capsule disintegration), purity, or compositional specifications, based on validated assay or other appropriate methods, that the supplement is represented to meet.".

(b) Supplement Listing on Nutrition Labeling. Section 403(q)(5)(F) (21 U.S.C. 343(q)(5)(F)) is amended to read as follows:

"(F) A dietary supplement product (including a food to which section 411 applies) shall comply with the requirements of subparagraphs (1) and (2) in a manner which is appropriate for the product and which is specified in regulations of the Secretary which shall provide that -

"(i) nutrition information shall first list those dietary ingredients that are present in the product in a significant amount and for which a recommendation for daily consumption has been established by the Secretary, except that a dietary ingredient shall not be required to be listed if it is not present in a significant amount, and shall list any other dietary ingredient present and identified as having no such recommendation;

"(ii) the listing of dietary ingredients shall include the quantity of each such ingredient (or of a proprietary blend of such ingredients) per serving;

"(iii) the listing of dietary ingredients may include the source of a dietary ingredient; and

"(iv) the nutrition information shall immediately precede the ingredient information required under subclause (i), except that no ingredient identified pursuant to subclause (i) shall be required to be identified a second time.".

(c) Percentage Level Claims. Section 403(r)(2) (21 U.S.C. 343(r)(2)) is amended by adding after clause (E) the following:

"(F) Subclause (i) clause (A) does not apply to a statement in the labeling of a dietary supplement that characterizes the percentage level of a dietary ingredient for which the Secretary has not established a reference daily intake, daily recommended value, or other recommendation for daily consumption.".

(d) Vitamins and Minerals. Section 411(b)(2) (21 U.S.C. 350(b)(2)) is amended -

(1) by striking "vitamins or minerals" and inserting "dietary supplement ingredients described in section 201(ff)";

(2) by striking "(2)(A)" and inserting "(2)"; and

(3) by striking subparagraph (B).

(e) Effective Date. Dietary supplements -

(1) may be labeled after the date of the enactment of this Act in accordance with the amendments made by this section, and

(2) shall be labeled after December 31, 1996, in accordance with such amendments.

§8. New Dietary Ingredients.
Chapter IV of the Federal Food, Drug, and Cosmetic Act is amended by adding at the end the following:

"NEW DIETARY INGREDIENTS

"**SEC. 413. (a) IN GENERAL.-** A dietary supplement which contains a new dietary ingredient shall be deemed adulterated under section 402(f) unless it meets one of the following requirements:

"(1) The dietary supplement contains only dietary ingredients which have been present in the food supply as an article used for food in a form in which the food has not been chemically altered.

"(2) There is a history of use or other evidence of safety establishing that the dietary ingredient when used under the conditions recommended or suggested in the labeling of the dietary supplement will reasonably be expected to be safe and, at least 75 days before being introduced or delivered for introduction into interstate commerce, the manufac-turer or distributor of the dietary ingredient or dietary supplement provides the Secretary with information, including any citation to published articles, which is the basis on which the manufacturer or distributor has concluded that a dietary supplement containing such dietary ingredient will reasonably be expected to be safe.

The Secretary shall keep confidential any information provided under paragraph (2) for 90 days following its receipt. After the expiration of such 90 days, the Secretary shall place such information on public display, except matters in the information which are trade secrets or otherwise confidential, commercial information.

"**(b) PETITION. -** Any person may file with the Secretary a petition proposing the issuance of an order prescribing the conditions under which a new dietary ingredient under its intended conditions of use will reasonably be expected to be safe. The Secretary shall make a decision on such petition within 180 days of the date the petition is filed with the Secretary. For purposes of chapter 7 of title 5, United States Code, the decision of the Secretary shall be considered final agency action.

"(c) **DEFINITION.** - For purposes of this section, the term "new dietary ingredient" means a dietary ingredient that was not marketed in the United States before October 15, 1994 and does not include any dietary ingredient which was marketed in the United States before October 15, 1994.".

§9. **Good Manufacturing Practices.**

Section 402 (21 U.S.C. 342), as amended by section 4, is amended by adding at the end the following:

"(g)(1) If it is a dietary supplement and it has been prepared, packed, or held under conditions that do not meet current good manufacturing practice regulations, including regulations requiring, when necessary, expiration date labeling, issued by the Secretary under subparagraph (2).

"(2) The Secretary may by regulation prescribe good manufacturing practices for dietary supplements. Such regulations shall be modeled after current good manufacturing practice regulations for food and may not impose standards for which there is no current and generally available analytical methodology. No standard of current good manufacturing practice may be imposed unless such standard is included in a regulation promulgated after notice and opportunity for comment in accordance with chapter 5 of title 5, United States Code.".

§10. Conforming Amendments.

(a) **SECTION 201** - The last sentence of section 201(g)(1) (21 U.S.C. 321(g)(1)) is amended to read as follows: "A food or dietary supplement for which a claim, subject to sections 403(r)(1)(B) and 403(r)(3) or sections 403(r)(1)(B) and 403(r)(5)(D), is made in accordance with the requirements of section 403(r) is not a drug solely because the label or the labeling contains such a claim. A food, dietary ingredient, or dietary supplement for which a truthful and not misleading statement is made in accordance with section 403(r)(6) is not a drug under clause (C) solely because the label or the labeling contains such a statement.".

(b) SECTION 301 - Section 301 (21 U.S.C. 331) is amended by adding at the end the following: (u) The introduction or delivery for introduction into interstate commerce of a dietary supplement that is unsafe under section 413.".

(c) SECTION 403 - Section 403 (21 U.S.C. 343), as amended by section 7, is amended by adding after paragraph (s) the following: "A dietary supplement shall not be deemed misbranded solely because its label or labeling contains directions or conditions of use or warnings.".

§11. Withdrawal of the Regulations and Notice.

The advance notice of proposed rulemaking concerning dietary supplements published in the Federal Register of June 18, 1993 (58 FR 33690-33700) is null and void and of no force or effect insofar as it applies to dietary supplements. The Secretary of Health and Human Services shall publish a notice in the Federal Register to revoke the item declared to be null and void and of no force or effect under subsection (a).

§12. Commission on Dietary Supplement Labels.

(a) ESTABLISHMENT. - There shall be established as an independent agency within the executive branch a commission to be known as the Commission on Dietary Supplement Labels (hereafter in this section referred to as the "Commission").

(b) MEMBERSHIP. -

(1) COMPOSITION. - The Commission shall be composed of 7 members who shall be appointed by the President.

(2) EXPERTISE REQUIREMENT. - The members of the Commission shall consist of individuals with expertise and experience in dietary supplements and in the manufacture, regulation, distribution, and use of such supplements. At least three of the members of the Commission shall be qualified by scientific training and experience to evaluate the benefits to health of the use

of dietary supplements and one of such three members shall have experience in pharmacognosy, medical botany, traditional herbal medicine, or other related sciences. Members and staff of the Commission shall be without bias on the issue of dietary supplements.

(c) FUNCTIONS OF THE COMMISSION. - The Commission shall conduct a study on, and provide recommendations for, the regulation of label claims and statements for dietary supplements, including the use of literature in connection with the sale of dietary supplements and procedures for the evaluation of such claims. In making such recommendations, **the Commission shall evaluate how best to provide truthful, scientifically valid, and not misleading information to consumers so that such consumers may make informed and appropriate health care choices for themselves and their families.**

(d) ADMINISTRATIVE POWERS OF THE COMMISSION. -
(1) HEARINGS. - The Commission may hold hearings, sit and act at such times and places, take such testimony, and receive such evidence as the Commission considers advisable to carry out the purposes of this section.
(2) INFORMATION FROM FEDERAL AGENCIES. - The Commission may secure directly from any Federal department or agency such information as the Commission considers necessary to carry out the provisions of this section.
(3) AUTHORIZATION OF APPROPRIATIONS. - There are authorized to be appropriated such sums as may be necessary to carry out this section.

(e) REPORTS AND RECOMMENDATIONS. -
(1) FINAL REPORT REQUIRED. - Not later than 24 months after the date of enactment of this Act, the Commission shall prepare and submit to the President and to the Congress a final report on the study required by this section.

(2) RECOMMENDATIONS. - The report described in paragraph (1) shall contain such recommendations, including recommendations for legislation, as the Commission deems appropriate.

(3) ACTION ON RECOMMENDATIONS. - Within 90 days of the issuance of the report under paragraph (1), the Secretary of Health and Human Services shall publish in the Federal Register a notice of any recommendation of Commission for changes in regulations of the Secretary for the regulation of dietary supplements and shall include in such notice a notice of proposed rulemaking on such changes together with an opportunity to present views on such changes. Such rulemaking shall be completed not later than 2 years after the date of the issuance of such report. If such rulemaking is not completed on or before the expiration of such 2 years, regulations of the Secretary published in 59 FR 395-426 on January 4, 1994, shall not be in effect.

§13. Office of Dietary Supplements.

(a) IN GENERAL. - Title IV of the Public Health Service Act is amended by inserting after section 485B (42 U.S.C. 287c-3) the following:

" **SUBPART 4--OFFICE OF DIETARY SUPPLEMENTS SEC. 485C. DIETARY SUPPLEMENTS.**

"(a) ESTABLISHMENT. - The Secretary shall establish an Office of Dietary Supplements within the National Institutes of Health.

"(b) PURPOSE. - The purposes of the Office are -

"(1) to explore more fully the potential role of dietary supplements as a significant part of the efforts of the United States to improve health care; and

"(2) to promote scientific study of the benefits of dietary supplements in maintaining health and preventing chronic disease and other health-related conditions.

"(c) DUTIES. - The Director of the Office of Dietary Supplements shall

    "(1) conduct and coordinate scientific research within the National Institutes of Health relating to dietary supplements and the extent to which the use of dietary supplements can limit or reduce the risk of diseases such as heart disease, cancer, birth defects, osteoporosis, cataracts, or prostatism;

    "(2) collect and compile the results of scientific research relating to dietary supplements, including scientific data from foreign sources or the Office of Alternative Medicine;

    "(3) serve as the principal advisor to the Secretary and to the Assistant Secretary for Health and provide advice to the Director of the National Institutes of Health, the Director of the Centers for Disease Control and Prevention, and the Commissioner of Food and Drugs on issues relating to dietary supplements including -

        "(A) dietary intake regulations;

        "(B) the safety of dietary supplements;

        "(C) claims characterizing the relationship between -

            "(i) dietary supplements; and

            "(ii)(I) prevention of disease or other health-related conditions; and

            "(II) maintenance of health; and

        "(D) scientific issues arising in connection with the labeling and composition of dietary supplements;

    "(4) compile a database of scientific research on dietary supplements and individual nutrients; and

    "(5) coordinate funding relating to dietary supplements for the National Institutes of

Health.

"(d) DEFINITION. - As used in this section, the term "dietary supplement" has the meaning given the term in section 201(ff) of the Federal Food, Drug, and Cosmetic Act.

"(e) AUTHORIZATION OF APPROPRIATIONS. - There are authorized to be appropriated to carry out this section $5,000,000 for fiscal year 1994 and such sums as may be necessary for each subsequent fiscal year.".

(b) CONFORMING AMENDMENT. - Section 401(b)(2) of the Public Health Service Act (42 U.S.C. 281(b)(2)) is amended by adding at the end the following:

"(E) The Office of Dietary Supplements.".

Approved October 25, 1994.

But, never funded.

Trust is Lacking Nearly Everywhere You Turn

The public breaks out in wild applaud at the drop of a criticism of Big Pharma especially from a politician. Trust in the integrity of the pharmaceutical industry is gone as they have come under increased scrutiny.

Our Texas Senator Ted Cruz, when he was on the presidential campaign trail, was often asked questions about healthcare and pharmaceutical companies. His answers began resinating with the people. But, Senator Cruz he took action that aligned with his words.

> *"We need to tear down the barriers blocking a new era of medical innovation, and the primary inhibitor is the government itself. It's past time to unleash a supply-side medical revolution, so that instead of simply caring for people with debilitating diseases, we cure them.*
>
> *"Beyond reforming reciprocity, we need to modernize the FDA's approach, expand the Accelerating Medicines Partnership (AMP), and embrace a culture of innovation, as foundations like XPrize are doing."*
>
> - Senator Ted Cruz

A Letter to the FDA Commissioner
Lax Regulation on Deadly Drugs is a Concern

Sen. Cruz and 74 Members of Congress
Demand Answers from FDA Commissioner

On Monday April 25, 2016 U.S. Senator Ted Cruz (R-Texas) joined 74 members of Congress in sending a letter to the FDA Commissioner Robert

Califf expressing serious concerns and demanded answers regarding the FDA's decision to loosen standards on the abortion drug Mifepristone.

In addition to killing the baby, serious harmful side effects are noted. Mifepristone is a prescription medication used to treat high blood sugar caused by high cortisol levels in the blood in adults with Cushing's syndrome and type 2 diabetes or glucose intolerance. However, one of the noted side effects is high blood pressure, headaches, nausea, fatigue, low potassium in your blood, pain in your arms and legs (arthralgia), vomiting, swelling of your arms and legs (peripheral edema) and dizziness. Mifepristone is a cortisol receptor blocker that blocks the actions of cortisol to lower blood sugar levels.

The letter to the FDA states that Congress is "deeply disappointed to learn that you have loosened FDA standards governing use of the abortion drug mifepristone, also referred to as Mifeprex or RU-486."

Mifepristone is associated with serious adverse events including hemorrhaging, severe infections and deaths of mothers who have taken it. The drug's original approval process was extremely controversial.

The letter express concerns about recent changes to the FDA-Approved Regimen and the Risk Evaluation and Mitigation Strategy (REMS) for Mifeprex (mifepristone) announced on March 30, 2016."

In addition to Senator Cruz, other signatures included the following members of Congress also signed onto the letter: Sen. Roy Blunt (R-Mo.), Sen. Steve Daines (R-Mont.), Sen. Joni Ernst (R-Iowa), Sen. James Lankford (R-Okla.), Sen. Mike Lee (R-Utah), Sen. Jerry Moran (R-Kan.), Sen. James Risch (R-Idaho), Sen. David Vitter (R-La.), Rep. Rick Allen (R-Ga.), Rep. Brian Babin (R-Texas), Rep. Dan Benishek (R-Mich.), Rep. Diane Black (R-Tenn.), Rep. Charles Boustany (R-La.), Rep. Kevin Brady (R-Texas), Rep. Dave Brat (R-Va.), Rep. Earl 'Buddy' Carter (R-Ga.), Rep. Steve Chabot (R-Ohio), Rep. Tom Cole (R-Okla.), Rep. Sean Duffy (R-Wis.), Rep. Jeff Duncan (R-S.C.), Rep. Blake Farenthold (R-Texas), Rep. John Fleming (R-La.), Rep. Bill Flores (R-Texas), Rep. Randy Forbes (R-Va.), Rep. Jeff Fortenberry (R-Neb.), Rep. Virginia Foxx (R-N.C.), Rep. Trent Franks (R-Ariz.), Rep. Bob Gibbs (R-Ohio), Rep. Bob Goodlatte (R-Va.), Rep. Gregg Harper (R-Miss.), Rep. Vicky Hartzler (R-Mo.), Rep. Jeb Hensarling (R-Texas), Rep. Jody Hice (R-Ga.), Rep. Richard Hudson (R-N.C.), Rep. Tim Huelskamp (R-Kan.), Rep. Bill Huizenga (R-Mich.), Rep. Bill Johnson (R-Ohio), Rep. Sam Johnson (R-Texas), Rep. Walter Jones (R-N.C.), Rep. David Joyce (R-Ohio), Rep. Mike Kelly (R-Pa.), Rep. Trent Kelly (R-Miss.), Rep. Steve King (R-Iowa), Rep. Doug LaMalfa (R-Calif.), Rep. Doug Lamborn (R-Colo.), Rep. Daniel Lipinski (D-Ill.), Rep. Barry Loudermilk (R-Ga.), Rep. Blaine Luetkemeyer (R-Mo.), Rep. Mark Meadows (R-N.C.), Rep. Jeff Miller (R-Fla.), Rep. Alex Mooney (R-W.Va.), Rep. Markwayne Mullin (R-Okla.), Rep. Tim Murphy (R-Pa.), Rep. Randy Neugebauer (R-Texas), Rep. Pete Olson (R-Texas), Rep. Steve Pearce (R-N.M.), Rep. Robert Pittenger (R-N.C.), Rep. Joe Pitts (R-Pa.), Rep. Mike Pompeo (R-Kan.), Rep. John Ratcliffe (R-Texas), Rep. Phil Roe (R-Tenn.), Rep. Todd Rokita (R-Ind.), Rep. Keith Rothfus (R-Pa.), Rep. David Rouzer (R-N.C.), Rep. Steve Russell (R-Okla.), Rep. Matt Salmon (R-Ariz.), Rep. Chris Smith (R-N.J.), Rep. Chris Stewart (R-Utah), Rep. Ann Wagner (R-Mo.), Rep. Tim Walberg (R-Mich.), Rep. Mark Walker (R-N.C.), Rep. Randy Weber (R-Texas), Rep. Daniel Webster (R-Fla.), and Rep. Kevin Yoder (R-Kan.).

114th CONGRESS
1ST SESSION

S. 2388

To amend the Federal Food, Drug, and Cosmetic Act to provide for reciprocal marketing approval of certain drugs, biological products, and devices that are authorized to be lawfully marketed abroad, and for other purposes.

IN THE SENATE OF THE UNITED STATES
DECEMBER 10, 2015

Mr. CRUZ (for himself and Mr. Lee) introduced the following bill; which was read twice and referred to the Committee on Health, Education, Labor, and Pensions

A BILL

To   amend the Federal Food, Drug, and Cosmetic Act to provide for reciprocal marketing approval of certain drugs, biological products, and devices that are authorized to be lawfully marketed abroad, and for other purposes.

1   *Be it enacted by the Senate and House of Representa-*
2   *tives of the United States of America in Congress*
       assembled,

3   **SECTION 1. Short title.**
4   This Act may be cited as the "Reciprocity Ensures
5   Streamlined Use of Lifesaving Treatments Act of 2015".

1 **SEC. 2. RECIPROCAL MARKETING APPROVAL FOR CERTAIN**
2   **DRUGS, BIOLOGICAL PRODUCTS, AND DE-**
3   **VICES.**
4 The Federal Food, Drug, and Cosmetic Act is amend-
5 ed by inserting after section 524A of such Act (21 U.S.C.
6 360n–1) the following:
7 **"SEC. 524B. Reciprocal marketing approval.**
8   "(a) IN GENERAL.—A covered product with recip-
9 rocal marketing approval in effect under this section is
10 deemed to be subject to an application or premarket notifi-
11 cation for which an approval or clearance is in effect under
12 section 505(c), 510(k), or 515 of this Act or section
13 351(a) of the Public Health Service Act, as applicable.
14 "(b) ELIGIBILITY.—The Secretary shall, with respect
15 to a covered product, grant reciprocal marketing approval
16 if—
17   "(1) the sponsor of the covered product submits
18 a request for reciprocal marketing approval; and
19   "(2) the request demonstrates to the Sec-
20 retary's satisfaction that—
21   "(A) the covered product is authorized to
22 be lawfully marketed in one or more of the
23 countries included in the list under section
24 802(b)(1);

1   "(B) absent reciprocal marketing approval,
2   the covered product is not approved or cleared
3   for marketing, as described in subsection (a);
4   "(C) the Secretary has not, because of any
5   concern relating to the safety or effectiveness of
6   the covered product, rescinded or withdrawn
7   any such approval or clearance;
8   "(D) the authorization to market the cov-
9   ered product in one or more of the countries in-
10   cluded in the list under section 802(b)(1) has
11   not, because of any concern relating to the safe-
12   ty or effectiveness of the covered product, been
13   rescinded or withdrawn;
14   "(E) the covered product is not a banned
15   device under section 516; and
16   "(F) there is a public health or unmet
17   medical need for the covered product in the
18   United States.
19   "(c) Safety and effectiveness.—
20   "(1) IN GENERAL.—The Secretary—
21   "(A) may decline to grant reciprocal mar-
22   keting approval under this section with respect
23   to a covered product if the Secretary affirma-
24   tively determines that the covered product—

1   "(i) is a drug that is not safe and ef-
2   fective; or
3   "(ii) is a device for which there is no
4   reasonable assurance of safety and effec-
5   tiveness; and
6   "(B) may condition reciprocal marketing
7   approval under this section on the conduct of
8   specified postmarket studies, which may include
9   such studies pursuant to a risk evaluation and
10 mitigation strategy under section 505–1.
11   "(2) REPORT TO CONGRESS.—Upon declining
12 to grant reciprocal marketing approval under this
13 section with respect to a covered product, the Sec-
14 retary shall—
15   "(A) include the denial in a list of such de-
16   nials for each month; and
17   "(B) not later than the end of the respec-
18   tive month, submit the list to the Committee on
19   Energy and Commerce of the House of Rep-
20   resentatives and the Committee on Health,
21   Education, Labor and Pensions of the Senate.
22 "(d) Request.—A request for reciprocal marketing
23 approval shall—
24   "(1) be in such form, be submitted in such
25 manner, and contain such information as the Sec-

1   retary deems necessary to determine whether the cri-
2   teria listed in subsection (b)(2) are met; and
3   "(2) include, with respect to each country in-
4   cluded in the list under section 802(b)(1) where the
5   covered product is authorized to be lawfully mar-
6   keted, as described in subsection (b)(2)(A), an
7   English translation of the dossier issued by such
8   country to authorize such marketing.
9   "(e) TIMING.—The Secretary shall issue an order
10 granting, or declining to grant, reciprocal marketing ap-
11 proval with respect to a covered product not later than
12 30 days after the Secretary's receipt of a request under
13 subsection (b)(1) for the product. An order issued under
14 this subsection shall take effect subject to Congressional
15 disapproval under subsection (g).
16 "(f) LABELING; DEVICE CLASSIFICATION.—During
17 the 30-day period described in subsection (e)—
18   "(1) the Secretary and the sponsor of the cov-
19 ered product shall expeditiously negotiate and final-
20 ize the form and content of the labeling for a cov-
21 ered product for which reciprocal marketing ap-
22 proval is to be granted; and
23   "(2) in the case of a device for which reciprocal
24 marketing approval is to be granted, the Secretary
25 shall—

1   "(A) classify the device pursuant to section
2   513; and
3   "(B) determine whether, absent reciprocal
4   marketing approval, the device would need to be
5   cleared pursuant to section 510(k) or approved
6   pursuant to section 515 to be lawfully marketed
7   under this Act.
8   "(g) CONGRESSIONAL DISAPPROVAL OF FDA OR-
9 DERS.—
10   "(1) IN GENERAL.—A decision of the Secretary
11 to decline to grant reciprocal marketing approval
12 under this section shall not take effect if a joint res-
13 olution of disapproval of the decision is enacted.
14   "(2) PROCEDURE.—
15   "(A) IN GENERAL.—Subject to subpara-
16   graph (B), the procedures described in sub-
17   sections (b) through (g) of section 802 of title
18   5, United States Code, shall apply to the con-
19   sideration of a joint resolution under this sub-
20   section.
21   "(B) TERMS.—For purposes of this sub-
22   section—
23   "(i) the reference to 'section
24   801(a)(1)' in section 802(b)(2)(A) of title

1	5, United States Code, shall be considered
2	to refer to subsection (c)(2); and
3	"(ii) the reference to 'section
4	801(a)(1)(A)' in section 802(e)(2) of title
5	5, United States Code, shall be considered
6	to refer to subsection (c)(2).
7	"(3) EFFECT OF CONGRESSIONAL DIS-
8	APPROVAL.—Reciprocal marketing approval under
9	this section with respect to the applicable covered
10	product shall take effect upon enactment of a joint
11	resolution of disapproval under this subsection.
12	"(h) APPLICABILITY OF RELEVANT PROVISIONS.—
13	The provisions of this Act shall apply with respect to a
14	covered product for which reciprocal marketing approval
15	is in effect to the same extent and in the same manner
16	as such provisions apply with respect to a product for
17	which approval or clearance of an application or pre-
18	market notification under section 505(c), 510(k), or 515
19	of this Act or section 351(a) of the Public Health Service
20	Act, as applicable, is in effect.
21	"(i) FEES FOR REQUEST.—For purposes of imposing
22	fees under chapter VII, a request for reciprocal marketing
23	approval under this section shall be treated as an applica-
24	tion or premarket notification for approval or clearance

1   under section 505(c), 510(k), or 515 of this Act or section
2   351(a) of the Public Health Service Act, as applicable.
3   "(j) OUTREACH.—The Secretary shall conduct an
4   outreach campaign to encourage the sponsors of covered
5   products that are potentially eligible for reciprocal mar-
6   keting approval to request such approval.
7   "(k) Covered product defined.—In this section,
8   the term 'covered product' means a drug, biological prod-
9   uct, or device.".

O

Never ever underestimate what you can do.

Chapter Ten

A Look in the Mirror

The FDA is not the Rat.

**Should we blame the drug companies'
for the medical chaos?**

**Should we blame the government
for the medical chaos?**

**Surely, it is not the fault of the doctors
for the medical chaos?**

"We have met the enemy and he is us." – Walt Kelly said, in his most famous cartoon character, Pogo, spoke his most famous recorded words.

The silent battle to mask symptoms has built the medical road on which we travel today. The central theme of medical and healthcare became *"Fix me, doctor."* The ever new miracle wonder drug enabled the doctor and patient to kick the can down the road of sickness.

Doctor and Patient Became Co-Dependent

Co-dependent on each other, the patient and doctor continued to skip down the road together. The patient, in-lieu-of accepting responsibility for his or her own health, paid the doctor to handle that responsibility. With each discomfort, the patient demanded another *"fix"* today. Drugs often met the need of the moment and the allopathic road was built. The road was paved with good intentions.

So, here we are, with a broken medical system based on the demands of the patient as though healthcare is a right instead of a responsibility. Like a cancer, the cry mutated from, *"Fix me now."* to "Fix me now because good health is my right. Then it metastasized, *"And, I want someone else to pay for it."*

The road we take, the habits we form, are triggered by how we respond or react. Human nature is to do whatever it takes to survive. Beyond the basic survival instinct is the immense crave for immediate self-gratification even when it is not urgent or perhaps not even important.

From the perspective of a diabetic, *"It is much easier to eat the donut than to not eat the donut."* It is more difficult to be proactive than to take the easy road of eating another donut. Responsibility is the right. Health is the choice for most people.

A wise response is based on intellectual integrity calculated for future success. A hasty reaction is based on the emotional need or desire of the moment. Our intent may be honorable – be it response or reaction. But, as we observe the medical landscape, the road to hell is paved with good intentions.

Immunology - Our Only Hope

Because of resistant bacteria and mutating viruses, many doctors and research scientists understand that we are about out of can and road.

In addition to man becoming his own worst enemy. Nobel laureate, Dr. Joshua Lederberg, has stated, "*Our only real competitors for dominion of the planet remain the viruses.*"

It is a time for results. It is time we seek the road of wellness by discovering the cause and effect and develop a common cure for all diseases. The cure is through immunology. Immunology is our natural prevention system. We are not to die sick. We are to live healthy lives on the road of wellness. We may all die but we do not have to die sick.

No More Finger Pointing

It is a time for truth, action, and results. Pointing fingers and blaming the FDA, the government, the drug companies, the doctors is going down the same road of chaos. The truth is that we have been on the road of sickness instead of wellness. The action each of us needs to take is to first look in the mirror and take a good look at the enemy.

There is no action required to battle the enemy of self nor anyone else. Just get on the right road. You will not be alone on this road of wellness. This is not an alternative route. This is not even a complementary route. This road of wellness is an integrative route and everyone is welcome to go this route and to bring their neighbors.

Integrating Glycoscience

Doctors will become better doctors and their patients will thank them and tell their neighbor how great is their doctor. For many years, my moto has been, "Whatever works the best and helps people the most and does no harm."

"Do no harm" will be brought back into the equation through Glycoscience. It is we the people who have driven the market for drugs. And, it is we the people who have been the enemy. And, it is we the people who must get on the road of wellness instead of the road of sickness.

It is we the people who must free ourselves from the tether of the FDA's LD_{50} rule.

Walt Kelly and his character, Pogo, would be proud that we have finally recognized who is the enemy.

To React or to Respond?

To be reactive or to be proactive?

To be proactive will shadow reactions and responses and prevent harm!

The next step is to learn more.
A people must have knowledge or they perish.

The next step then is to act on the education.

Chapter Eleven

What Can The People Do Now?

Education

To educate yourself in the science of the sugars will enable you to make better health decisions. Understand that without knowledge, the people perish. A friend said to me, *"Glycoscience education is the second most important message that must be taken to the world."*

Since 1996, I have studied the works of over 700 M.D.s, PhDs, Scientists, Researchers, and Educators in the field of Glycoscience and brain function and collaborated with schools, universities, or research labs in thirteen countries.

Leading scientists had scoffed at the work of several of my friends and cohorts. The scoffers declared their research was not science at all and that improving glycosylation of the human cell was impossible. A Texas R&D company in 2011 funded an open label study that concluded that improved glycosylation is possible.

In 2012, the National Academies published through the National Academies Press *Transforming Glycoscience - A Road Map for the Future*. A distinguished panel of glycoscientists was commissioned for a collaborative effort to explore the future of Glycoscience. The National Research Council drew from the National Academies: the National Academy of Sciences, National Academy of Engineering, Institute of Medicine. The project was supported by National Institutes of Health, the National Science Foundation, U.S. Department of Energy, the Food and Drug Administration, and the Howard Hughes Medical Institute. Together, they were commissioned to develop the roadmap for the future of Glycoscience.

The report contained profound statements including:

"Glycans impact the structure/function of every living cell in humans, animals, and plants."

The Academy expanded on the importance of the sugars, saying:

"Glycans play roles in almost every biological process and are involved in every major disease" and
"Elimination of any single class of glycans from an organism results in death."

The GLYCOSCIENCE INSTITUTE in Houston

The GLYCOSCIENCE INSTITUTE in Houston was founded in 2016 for the purpose of providing basic Glycoscience education to physicians, all healthcare professions, and the general public.

The mission of the GLYCOSCIENCE INSTITUTE is to continually compile scientific information that can be easily understood even for the layperson. This is achieved by collaborating with universities and research groups in many countries to stay current with developments.

The National Library of Medicine has recorded some 700,000 references that point to research already conducted on some of the most significant life changing biological sugars. The majority of these papers were published within the last few years.

You may request a free Update Report from the GLYCOSCIENCE INSTITUTE
http://GlycoScienceInstitute.com

The TEXAS ENDOWMENT FOR MEDICAL RESEARCH

The TEXAS ENDOWMENT FOR MEDICAL RESEARCH was founded as a nonprofit faith-based organization in 2017 for the purpose of collaborating with researchers to conduct Pilot Studies to improve glycosylation. With the focus on glycosylation, regardless of the patient's health challenge, the results are self-evident without treating or curing any disease.

Foundations, corporations, organizations, small co-ops, and the general public may participate through Crowd Funding, Grant Writing, and general contribution to sponsor a friend or family member into a specific recovery program. The TEXAS ENDOWMENT FOR MEDICAL RESEARCH will attempt to match funding for any health challenge when gathering clinical data.

You may request a free Update Report from the TEXAS ENDOWMENT FOR MEDICAL RESEARCH　　　　http://TexasEndowment.com

Ten Ways You Can Make a Difference in Your World

Example: Take one major health issue with which you are familiar or for which you have a passion. Know anyone with PTSD, diabetes, Alzheimer's, Parkinson's or another significant health challenge?

Form a team of two or more. A team, a club, or group is simply made up of caring individuals linked together. Together, involve friends and family with the intent of helping someone within or outside the group.

Organize a **Crowd Funding Project** or a **Pay It Forward Project** and ask a friend to help you. Seek out a veteran with a health challenge, especially if it is neurological. Sponsor them into a Pilot Survey where a doctor of their choice can monitor their improvement. Matched funding is available.

Download Free Report "**Ten Ways to Kill A Rat and Make A Difference in Your World.**"　　　　http://ToKillARatBook.com

More than Just for Today

The information we gather today through our Pilot Studies will potentially impact many live in the future and possibly eliminate some health challenges along the way.

The Future is Bright but Expect Challenges and Complications

As we overcome challenges and complications we make new discoveries and have greater results.

Our purpose in life is to help others worse off than ourselves. As we pay it forward, as we help others, money will be no problem. Health is the bigger issue.

It is A Time for Truth. It is A Time for Action. It is Time for RESULTS.

We overcome our personal challenges as we overcome the old mind set. The old mind set is that it may be too heard or impossible. This results in under performing. The under-performance mind set is well described by "fleas in a jar." Fleas can jump a hundred times their height. But you can train a flea to underperform. To train a flea put him in a jar and let him hit his little head on the lid enough times until he is conditioned. Now, take the lid off and jar and he will continue to jump no higher than where the lid was.

A similar under-performance comparison is to put a rope on a baby elephant's leg tied to a stake to keep it tethered and controlled. When the elephant is an adult, the tether still holds and controls .

We have been tethered by the FDA's LD_{50} rule for nearly a century. It is time to break the tether.

True stories of hope where there was no hope.

To Kill A Rat

The FDA requires millions of animals to die to develop new drugs.

You want your doctor to "*Do no harm!*" but the medical battle cry of yesteryear was lost to toxic drugs. The FDA uses an antiquated LD_{50} criteria for drug approval. The LD_{50} standard was established to measure just how harmful is any medicine. Lethal Dose 50 requires that all new drugs must kill 50 percent of the subjects in animal studies. Any medicine that cannot establish a LD_{50} level is ruled out from any consideration for FDA approval. This single procedure eliminates the toxin free cures from ever reaching the market.

During the last century, the focus has been on problems instead of solutions. The medical industry addresses the immediate symptom instead of finding a cure. The drug establishment knows that the more critical and widespread the problem, the greater the opportunity for profit. The focus remains on sickness instead of wellness.

"We need to tear down the barriers blocking a new era of medical innovation, and the primary inhibitor is the government itself. It's past time to unleash a supply-side medical revolution, so that instead of simply caring for people with debilitating diseases, we cure them. ... and embrace a culture of innovation"

- Senator Ted Cruz

No rat was injured or killed in the writing of this book.

The U.S. Department of Agriculture (USDA) compiles annual statistics on the number of animals including dogs, cats, primates, rabbits, hamsters, guinea pigs, and other animals used in research in the United States. The Humane Society of the United States estimates that more than twenty-five million (25,000,000) vertebrate animals are used annually in research, testing, and education in the United States. This practice has continued for nearly a century. This book is not a campaign to save animals nor is it an effort to justify torturing and killing animals in the name of science. Rather, the book is a testament for how unnecessary is the FDA's LD_{50} mandate **To Kill A Rat**.

Made in the USA
San Bernardino, CA
25 March 2017